CARLTON FREDERICKS'
GUIDE TO
WOMEN'S NUTRITION

ALSO BY CARLTON FREDERICKS

Carlton Fredericks' Sodium Counter
New Low Blood Sugar and You
Low Blood Sugar and You
Look Younger, Feel Healthier
Carlton Fredericks' Low Carbohydrate Diet
Carlton Fredericks' Cookbook for Good Nutrition
The Low Blood Sugar Cookbook
Psychonutrition
Winning the Fight Against Breast Cancer
Eat Well, Stay Well
Arthritis: You Don't Have to Learn to Live With It

CARLTON FREDERICKS' GUIDE TO WOMEN'S NUTRITION

by Carlton Fredericks, Ph.D.

Compiled and edited by Carol-June Cassidy

A PERIGEE BOOK

Perigee Books
are published by
The Putnam Publishing Group
200 Madison Avenue
New York, NY 10016

First Perigee Edition 1989
Copyright © 1988 by The Estate of Dr. Carlton Fredericks
All rights reserved. This book, or parts thereof,
may not be reproduced in any form without permission.
Published simultaneously in Canada

Acknowledgments:
    The Estate of Carlton Fredericks, Ph.D., for material from *Winning the Fight Against Breast Cancer* by Carlton Fredericks, Ph.D., copyright © 1977 by Carlton Fredericks, Ph.D.
    Grosset & Dunlap for material from *Carlton Fredericks' New Low Blood Sugar and You,* copyright © 1969, © 1985 by Carlton Fredericks.

Library of Congress Cataloging-in-Publication Data

Fredericks, Carlton.
    [Guide to women's nutrition]
    Carlton Fredericks' guide to women's nutrition / by Carlton Fredericks; compiled and edited by Carol-June Cassidy.—1st Perigee ed.

        p.   cm.
    Reprint. Originally published: New York: Putnam, © 1988.
    Includes index.
    1. Women—Health and hygiene—Popular works.   2. Women—Nutrition—Popular works.   3. Women—Diseases—Prevention—Popular works.   I. Cassidy, Carol-June, date.   II. Title.   III. Title: Guide to women's nutrition.
[RA778.F856   1989]
618.1'0654—dc20
ISBN 0-399-51571-2   89-3895 CIP

Printed in the United States of America
1   2   3   4   5   6   7   8   9   10

CONTENTS

1 | NUTRITION AND HEALTH

If I ask a group of average Americans if they are healthy, I hear: "Yes, I'm healthy. I have a little sinus trouble . . . a little postnasal drip . . . a little indigestion . . . a little heartburn . . . a little constipation . . . a few allergies . . . my circulation's a bit poor . . . I have dandruff . . . my hair is dry . . . but I'm healthy."

What does this mean? It means: "I don't have cancer, thank heavens . . . or TB . . . or heart disease . . . or hardening of the arteries." I had a young woman come to see me once. She had nothing "wrong" with her. She wasn't sick, but she didn't feel truly well. She wanted her diet and supplements straightened out while she was still reasonably healthy.

Nutrition is polypharmaceutical, which is to say that one nutrient relates to another and those relate to a third, and the third to a fourth—isolated nutrients should not be prescribed because of the importance of these interactions. I complied with her request and she dropped me a line some time later saying she never knew before what it was like to feel wonderful. Unfortunately, you don't get her kind of request very often. This is sad, since the name of the game is prevention.

I can think of only one vitamin that was introduced without controversy from the medical establishment: vitamin K. Other vitamins have been surrounded by controversy from the beginning: thiamine, vitamin B_3, vitamin C, vitamin E, pyridoxine. Riboflavin, vitamin B_{12}, and folic acid largely escaped controversy, though I don't know why. The irrational acceptance or rejection of vitamins is intrinsic to orthodox medicine, which has always been conservative: Be not the first to lay the old aside nor the first to adopt the new. This set of contradictions engenders nothing but mental constipation and complete resistance to innovation. Orthodox medicine does not teach its graduates its own history, so they do not realize that today's orthodox treatment was rejected yesterday as quackery. Perhaps if medical students were given courses in the history and philosophy of medicine they would be more open to new ideas and the time it now takes to go from heresy to orthodoxy would be shortened.

Medicine pays more attention to theory than to observation. The medical establishment often does not seem aware that theories change. They are altered with each new fact that is picked up through observation. But observations are permanent, and the facts of medicine are observations. The Chinese knew four thousand years ago that liver (a source of vitamin A) helps eyesight at night; it was known tens of decades ago that vitamin A is involved in eyesight, yet medicine didn't catch up with the fact until comparatively recently.

A new set of observations that runs afoul of established orthodox thinking is called a new paradigm. New paradigms in medicine are almost always rejected at first. There is always a series of hard-fought battles and then the new ideas take root, eventually displacing the old ideas. The new ideas become the new orthodoxy, and that new orthodoxy rejects the next innovation.

The vitamins have been involved in a number of new paradigms. Up to the time they were discovered, disease was thought always to be caused by the *presence* of something—a "germ," for example.

Then vitamins began to be better understood, and with that came the concept that disease could be caused by the *absence* of something. This notion turned the medical world upside down. The absence of something as a cause of disease was too alien a concept; it promptly delayed acceptance of vitamins. Eventually a new orthodoxy arose: Doctors accepted the new concept, but they went on to say vitamins were required only for deficiency diseases. In other words, if you did not have beriberi, scurvy, pellagra, or rickets you were not vitamin deficient and vitamins could not do anything for you; moreover, only the minute doses that would prevent those diseases of deficiency were needed.

FACTORS PREDISPOSING TO VITAMIN DEFICIENCY*

Inadequate Intake. Due to poverty, ignorance, working conditions, availability of foods, cultural patterns, fad diets, gastrointestinal disorders (e.g., anorexia, bulimia), chronic alcoholism, advanced age, prolonged intravenous glucose infusion, restricted diets (including infant formula), neuropsychiatric disorders, pregnancy.

Impaired Absorption. Due to gastrointestinal disorders, excessive use of mineral oil, cardiovascular disease, advanced age, infant prematurity and feeding problems.

Inadequate Utilization or Storage. Due to diabetes, diseases of the kidney, liver, or pancreas, hypothyroidism, antibiotic therapy, malignancy.

Increased Requirement. Due to hyperthyroidism, physical exertion, pregnancy and lactation, rapid growth, infection and fever, surgical treatment, injury, burns, and convalescence.

Increased Loss or Excretion. Caused by blood loss, polyuria, negative nitrogen balance, lactation.

*Adapted from *American Practitioner*, vol. 13, no. 8 (August 1962), p. 19A.

So we see that the concept of vitamins was accepted by medicine gradually and then became fossilized, preventing the proper examination of vitamin therapy for a large number of diseases. This is only now beginning to change slowly.

In a study that clearly showed the effects of inadequate nutrient intake, 260 noninstitutionalized elderly people were tested on memory and abstract thinking ability. It was found that those with the lowest intake of nutrients and lowest blood levels of nutrients did not do well on the tests. Their test scores were within the normal limits, but those who ate less well functioned less well mentally. The specific nutrient deficiencies that interfered with mental function were: low dietary intake of protein, vitamins C, B_1, B_2, B_6, niacin, and folic acid; low blood levels of vitamins C, B_2, B_6, B_{12}, and folic acid. But neither the intake nor the blood levels were low enough to be considered clinically nutrient deficient. This was an attack of inferior nutrition on the ability of the brain to function without any visible physical signs of trouble in the body. Furthermore, all these people were getting the RDA of niacin and 90 percent of them were getting the RDA in vitamin C.

One of the things that happens as you grow older is that you get locked into a pattern of eating that becomes ever more rigid as the years go by—more and more difficult to leave behind or alter. Unfortunately, the person who resists a change in diet will usually also resist taking a vitamin supplement. In addition, the sense of smell and the sense of taste become less acute as you grow older. There's no pleasure in trying something new if you can't taste it, or savor it fully. (I have seen patients who had lost their sense of taste and smell completely or in whom it had become bizarrely distorted, so that things that normally would taste good tasted horrible to them and odors that are normally pleasant became intolerable. That can happen in pregnancy, and I have a hunch that when a woman exhibits that, she needs more zinc in her diet. If she doesn't get it not only will her sense of taste be distorted, but she will be more subject to stretch marks.)

There are always individual differences in nutritional tolerances, and requirements and individual differences exist in many other areas as well. You have only to watch two different people in the dentist's chair to realize how different the threshold for pain is from one person to another. It is fascinating to realize too that we can raise that threshold with nutrients so that people who ordinarily are very sensitive become less so or even remark that they are free of pain entirely. This can be done nutritionally for migraine headache, arthritis, and many other painful disorders.

There are "authorities" who will tell you that the way to nutritional salvation is to eat peas and beans and grains. Some vegetarians say that protein, which is the dominant constituent of our bodies, is poisonous. Others believe you can live on fruit alone. Each is convinced that he has the monopoly on truth. But there is only one food on the face of the earth to which we can point with certainty and say: "This was intended for consumption by humans." That food is breast milk. Now beyond breast milk everything is guess work.

On average, in a year you eat approximately 1402 pounds of food; 35 tons in a lifetime. That's a terrible figure, and it gives you one.

We live in a violent society. Unfortunately, the interpretation of that violence is monopolized by the behavioral psychologists, who tell us our children are raised without hope, no jobs, poor surroundings, poor playmates, too much peer pressure. Yet these fancy explanations overlook the fact that the kind of food eaten by pregnant women can adversely affect the child. Indeed, the kind of food eaten throughout our society disturbs the brain and the nervous system and is conducive to hostile, aggressive, socially undesirable, violent behavior. The penal system goes on operating blind to this fact, and the psychologists also refuse to look at it.

The types of food we eat, and the lack of essential nutrients in them due to overprocessing, contribute greatly to women's health

13

problems—particularly those caused by poor control of the female hormone estrogen: premenstrual syndrome, cystic mastitis, endometriosis, uterine fibroids, breast cancer. In the 1940s I came to the realization that the process which causes premenstrual symptoms, the process which makes the average American woman's menstrual history abnormal, is one that can come under dietary control.

Control of estrogen is a nutritional process. The hormone needs to be regulated, whether you are taking it by prescription or manufacturing it yourself, in which case it is regulated by the liver. The liver must deal with the hormone or you are in danger. Excessive intake of sugar and inadequate intake of protein and vitamin B complex will prevent the liver from doing its job. A five-day menstrual period is average, but if you use less sugar and eat adequate protein and increase your intake of vitamin B complex the period frequently drops to three days. I'm convinced five days is average, but it's not normal. Furthermore, it is evidence of a process that can lead to estrogen-dependent cancer.

Sugar

The label says sugar, then it says dextrose or glucose, then it says corn syrup or high-fructose corn syrup or fructose—it's all sugar, the ingredient present in the highest percentage for many foods.

There is no physiological requirement for sugar. Every nutritional need can be met in full without having a single spoonful of white, brown, or raw sugar. John Yudkin, former professor of biochemistry at Queen Elizabeth College in London, has said that if only a small fraction of what is already known about the effects of sugar were examined in relation to any other material used as a food additive, sugar would have to be banned.

Sugar now makes up about 25 percent of your calories. I'm going to give you a little idea what that does to you. In order to utilize a thousand calories from sugar, you need a half milligram of vitamin B_1 and proportionate amounts of riboflavin and niacinamide and a supply of chromium. But the sugar doesn't supply these vitamins and minerals. In fact, sugar causes you to excrete chromium. Magnesium deficiency in people on high-sugar diets is almost routine. It's hard enough to get adequate magnesium without a lot of sugar in the diet interfering with the intake of other foods. The sugar uses up your vitamin and mineral reserves and doesn't replenish them; it displaces the foods that could supply them. It's a parasite food.

There are patients whose gout becomes worse when they eat sugar; there is a relationship between sugar and rheumatoid arthritis; there is a relationship between sugar and cancer, in particular breast cancer (see chapter 4). There's another action attributable to sugar about which very few people know anything, and that is the action that causes myopia, nearsightedness. The proof is indirect: It has been noticed that when diabetics are not under good control—their blood sugar not kept at as near a normal level as possible—they tend to become slightly nearsighted.

In my experience, the greatest single cause of chronic indigestion is excessive sugar consumption. Indigestion keeps a large industry going in this country. While the medical establishment is complaining about the public "wasting" money on natural foods and vitamins, there are people who buy five hundred dollars' worth of antacid medication a month. Many of these antacids contain aluminum. I think this is a prime reason for the accumulation of high levels of aluminum in the brain, which is suspected of contributing to the development of Alzheimer's disease. (There are antacid preparations on the market that are a calcium source. Tums is an example, and I'm sure you can find others. I would prefer those to an aluminum source, because many women need more calcium.)

When you take in too much sugar, it displaces food that supplies

15

DISTRIBUTION OF SUGAR IN COMMON FOODS
(100 grams = 20 teaspoonfuls = 3½ ounces = 400 calories)

Food	Amount	Serving	Sugar Equivalent
Candy:			
Hershey bar	60 gm.	1 (25¢ size)	7 tsp. sugar
Chocolate cream	13 gm.	1 (35 to lb.)	2 tsp. sugar
Chocolate fudge	30 gm.	1½ in. sq. (15 to 1 lb.)	4 tsp. sugar
Chewing gum		1 stick	⅓ tsp. sugar
Lifesaver		1 usual size	⅓ tsp. sugar
Cake:			
Chocolate cake	100 gm.	2-layer, icing (1/12 cake)	15 tsp. sugar
Angel cake	45 gm.	1 pc. (1/12 large cake)	6 tsp. sugar
Sponge cake	50 gm.	1/10 of average cake	6 tsp. sugar
Cream puff (iced)	80 gm.	1 average, custard-filled	5 tsp. sugar
Doughnut (plain)	40 gm.	3 in. in diameter	4 tsp. sugar
Cookies:			
Macaroons	25 gm.	1 large or 2 small	3 tsp. sugar
Gingersnaps	6 gm.	1 medium	1 tsp. sugar
Brownies	20 gm.	2x2x¾ in.	3 tsp. sugar
Custards:			
Custard, baked		½ cup	4 tsp. sugar
Gelatin		½ cup	4 tsp. sugar
Junket		⅛ qt.	3 tsp. sugar
Soft drinks:			
Coca-Cola	180 gm.	1 bottle, 6 oz.	4⅓ tsp. sugar
Ginger ale	180 gm.	6-oz. glass	4⅓ tsp. sugar
Cooked fruits:			
Peaches, canned in syrup	10 gm.	2 halves, 1 Tbs. juice	3½ tsp. sugar
Rhubarb, stewed	100 gm.	½ cup, sweetened	8 tsp. sugar
Applesauce (no sugar)	100 gm.	½ cup, scant	2 tsp. sugar
Prunes, stewed, sweetened	100 gm.	4 to 5 medium	8 tsp. sugar

Dried fruits:

Item	Weight	Measure	Sugar equivalent
Apricots, dried	30 gm.	4 to 6 halves	4 tsp. sugar
Prunes, dried	30 gm.	3 to 4 medium	4 tsp. sugar
Dates, dried	30 gm.	3 to 4, stoned	4½ tsp. sugar
Figs, dried	30 gm.	1½ to 2 small	4 tsp. sugar
Raisins	30 gm.	¼ cup	4 tsp. sugar

Fruits and fruit juices:

Item	Weight	Measure	Sugar equivalent
Fruit cocktail	120 gm.	½ cup, scant	5 tsp. sugar
Orange juice	100 gm.	½ cup, scant	2 tsp. sugar
Pineapple juice, unsweetened	100 gm.	½ cup, scant	2⅗ tsp. sugar
Grapefruit juice, unsweetened	100 gm.	½ cup, scant	2⅕ tsp. sugar
Grape juice, commercial	100 gm.	½ cup, scant	3⅔ tsp. sugar

Ice cream:

Item	Measure	Sugar equivalent
Ice cream	⅛ qt.	5 to 6 tsp. sugar
Sherbet	⅛ qt.	6 to 8 tsp. sugar

Pie:

Item	Measure	Sugar equivalent
Apple pie	⅙ medium pie	12 tsp. sugar
Cherry pie	⅙ medium pie	14 tsp. sugar
Custard, coconut pie	⅙ medium pie	10 tsp. sugar
Pumpkin pie	⅙ medium pie	10 tsp. sugar

Sauce:

Item	Weight	Measure	Sugar equivalent
Chocolate sauce	30 gm.	1 heaping tsp., thick	4½ tsp. sugar
Marshmallow	7.6 gm.	1 (60 to 1 lb.)	1½ tsp. sugar

Spreads:

Item	Weight	Measure	Sugar equivalent
Jam	20 gm.	1 Tbs. level or 1 heaping tsp.	3 tsp. sugar
Jelly	20 gm.	1 Tbs. level or 1 heaping tsp.	2½ tsp. sugar
Marmalade	20 gm.	1 Tbs. level or 1 heaping tsp.	3 tsp. sugar
Honey	20 gm.	1 Tbs. level or 1 heaping tsp.	3 tsp. sugar

Milk drinks:

Item	Measure	Sugar equivalent
Chocolate (all milk)	1 cup, 5 oz. milk	6 tsp. sugar
Cocoa (all milk)	1 cup, 5 oz. milk	4 tsp. sugar
Cocomalt (all milk)	1 glass, 8 oz. milk	4 tsp. sugar

nutrients sugar doesn't supply—which is very easy, as sugar doesn't supply anything. And, what is removed from sugar—blackstrap molasses, for instance—is used to feed cattle.

I'm not trying to drive sugar out of your diet altogether. I can't. Not when tomato catsup is 20 percent sugar, a glazed doughnut contains seven teaspoons of sugar, and a portion of apple pie has twelve! I can't drive it out of your diet, and I wouldn't try. But I am trying to get it down to a reasonable amount. But I can assure those women who fight the battle of the bulge that if you take a hundred pounds of sugar out of your diet and don't replace it with anything, you should lose about thirty pounds in one year—while saving money too.

It is necessary to reorient your approach in order to reduce sugar intake. The quantities of sugar you are accustomed to should be reduced a bit at a time. If you make a cake at home and the recipe calls for two cups of sugar, cut it down by an eighth of a cup, then the next time by a quarter of a cup. There will come a point where the amount of sugar in a recipe cannot be reduced any further because the sugar is not only used for sweetness but also for texture. You will ultimately establish that point. Concentration wreaks havoc on your tastebuds for sugar. So the process must be gradual, but it can be accomplished and there are dividends beyond what you know.

The enormous intake of sugars and processed starches in the American diet has contributed to the problems caused by lack of fiber. The BAMBY plan (Bran And Multiple vitamins and minerals, B-complex vitamins—brewer's yeast or wheat germ or a concentrate—and Yogurt) is a combination of sensible diet and dietary factors that can prevent some of the troubles that accrue from lack of fiber, the wrong kind of bacterial flora, or lack of sufficient B-complex vitamins. We bring up the intake of fiber, we supply vitamins and minerals important to the functioning of the intestines, and we use plain, unflavored yogurt, sometimes fortified with freeze-dried lactobacillus acidophilus, to change bacterial flora to the friendly type.

You can't go out and just start using bran enthusiastically—you can get into trouble. It must be done gradually. Also, you don't start on bran and then suddenly stop. If you stop abruptly, you will develop the grandfather of all cases of constipation! Some safeguards are necessary.

Protein

Protein efficiency is determined on the basis of how much of the protein source is needed to maintain growth in the young child and to maintain the body's nitrogen balance. The nitrogen that comes into the body and the nitrogen being excreted should be in balance. If you excrete more nitrogen than you are taking in, you are tearing down the body's structure. That, incidentally, is what happens when you go on a fast. You go into negative nitrogen balance. Fasting is not a good method of weight reduction because it burns tissue, not fat.

You can always measure the nutritional quality of a protein by a simple criterion: The nearer the composition of a food is to your own composition, the more efficient it is. You are not made of vegetables or cereal, and you will find them low down on the list of useful protein. No vegetable protein, including soy, is equivalent to an animal protein.

As you go down this list, keep in mind that preceding proteins should be eaten with those that follow. The superior protein efficiency of one item, for instance eggs, will lift the protein efficiency of the next item, dairy, if they are served together. The same thing happens if the eggs or dairy product is served with an item farther down the list, such as meat or legumes. Each preceding protein, being biologically more efficient, helps you utilize the lesser proteins.

- EGGS. The most efficient protein. You can use less of eggs than any other protein to maintain growth and to keep nitrogen intake and output balanced.
- DAIRY. Milk, yogurt, and cheese are the protein source second highest in efficiency. In addition, they provide the calcium women need to avoid osteoporosis in their later years.
- MEAT, FISH, AND FOWL. It's hard for most Americans to believe that a piece of fish is nutritionally equivalent to a steak, but it is and it's better for you.
- LEGUMES. Peas and beans (including soybeans). Vegetarians take note: Soy protein is said to be equivalent to animal protein. It isn't. The soy on the market has been processed in a number of ways and this has had an adverse impact on its nutritional value. Also, soy interferes with zinc metabolism and, like all vegetable proteins, does not supply vitamin B_{12}.
- GRAINS. Least efficient of protein sources for two reasons: They have been treated with excessive heat; they generally do not contain enough of the amino acid lysine, which argues for combining different types of proteins. In the same way that a more efficient protein will lift the efficiency of a lesser protein source, sometimes by combining different grains one grain will make up for what is lacking in the next.

Two-thirds of the protein you eat, after you've satisfied your protein need from the other third (assuming your protein intake is adequate), is used as glucose. It's converted into fuel. The advantage of ingesting protein over the usual sources of glucose—carbohydrate starches and sugars—is that it is absorbed and metabolized more slowly. It provides lasting energy as opposed to the quick surge energy that results in an equally sudden "crash" and fatigue.

Caffeine

It is wise to eliminate use of caffeine-containing beverages. A chemical—xanthine—in caffeine can cause the development of cysts in the breasts. Not all breast cysts are so affected by caffeine, but some women will find relief if they discontinue the use of caffeine. It's certainly worth a try.

If there is any single cause of disturbances in the rhythm of the heart (other than heart disease), caffeine is it. We dose ourselves with it in many forms—cola and other soft drinks, tea, coffee, cocoa, chocolate, and over-the-counter drugs such as cold remedies and stimulants. People who get cardiac arrhythmias from caffeine are not necessarily consuming tremendous quantities of coffee, cola drinks, or whatever. Some are merely extremely sensitive to caffeine and as little as two hundred milligrams—about the amount in two cups of strong coffee—can touch off arterial flutter fibrillation, which may be dangerous, or ventricular tachycardia (rapid beating of the heart), which is less dangerous. Dangerous or not, it's disturbing.

A lot of mischief is caused by the amount of caffeine people consume. The percentage of patients who complain of cardiac arrhythmias is amazing. These arrhythmias range from meaningless skipped beats to abnormally slow beating to abnormally fast beating to sudden outbursts of abnormalities that may have serious meaning. (Skipped beats, by the way, are not really skipped. Sometimes one of the chambers of the heart pumps before it is full—that's called a PVB, or premature ventricular beat—and so then there is a longer gap than usual before the next beat.)

Too much caffeine—along with too much sugar and too much stress—induces panic attacks and hypoglycemia (see chapter 8), which can in turn trigger food allergies. Hypoglycemia—low blood sugar—can be identified and treated with a controlled diet, as I have described in detail in my book *Carlton Fredericks' New Low Blood Sugar and You,* and yet has often resulted in wasted time and

21

money spent in the psychiatrist's office. Though it can be controlled nutritionally, hypoglycemia's symptoms are often treated (or rather, left untreated) by orthodox medical practitioners as imagined, psychosomatic, hysterical complaints.

Psychiatric Misdiagnosis

I can't help thinking of the manner in which psychiatry approaches problems. The psychiatrist will not talk to a pregnant woman about the vitamin B_6 deficiency that is possibly causing her morning nausea. Instead he will ask questions intending to probe the woman's emotional state, attempting to reveal that she is trying to upchuck a baby she doesn't want.

How many patients referred for psychiatric care actually need a good internist? How many people who are accused of a mental, nervous, or emotional disorder actually have a physical disease that is either responsible for all their symptoms or worsens some of them? Some years ago on the West Coast, a team of internists took 115 patients diagnosed with psychiatric disorders and gave them careful physical exams. The results showed that all the patients had physical diseases that were responsible for their apparent mental symptoms; 5 of them had cancers and died within two years. In another study, 41 percent of the patients admitted to a psychiatric clinic with diagnoses of functional disorders were found to suffer from a physical disorder, and the medications they took, prescribed by their former doctors, caused many of their psychiatric symptoms. When an elderly person is placed under stress the risk of a mistaken psychiatric diagnosis is particularly great.

There are a great many women who are mistakenly diagnosed as neurotic or psychotic—more frequently neurotic—because they're tired, listless, their spirits are low, they've lost interest in things, are susceptible to infection, have multiple allergies. They wind up being sent home with a tranquilizer or antidepressant by their internist or begin analysis, treated by psychiatrists. The real *physical* problems they may be suffering from—hypoglycemia, body-wide yeast infection, mercury poisoning, premenstrual syndrome—are overlooked. They may be irritable, depressed due to intolerance of birth-control pills or doses of cortisone or prednisone or antibiotics prescribed for them that now contribute to the multiple allergies, candida infection, or chemical hypersensitivity they are suffering from.

Prevention

There is a whole list of chemical, drug, food, and environmental sensitivities people are bothered by (see chapter 5), and sometimes it is very difficult to separate and identify what the person is sensitive to. Is it tea? Is it the sugar you put in the tea? Is it the milk or cream you put in the tea? Or is it the slight amount of formaldehyde in the paper of the tea bag? Perhaps this is one of the reasons the medical establishment fights so hard against preventive approaches to health problems. In the field of allergy, this business of recognizing environmental influences is alternative—it is not practiced by all allergists by a long shot. The establishment would have to turn everything upside down, from taking the formaldehyde out of tea bags to a thousand other areas where we are chemically threatened. For those who suffer from chemical hypersensitivity we give antioxidants, the same antioxidants used to bolster the immune system and offset the side effects to chemotherapy and irradiation cancer treatments (see chapter 4).

Generally speaking, people whose diets are high in antioxidants tend to be younger than their years. I would rather you have in your diet the nutrients that are antidotes for oxidizing radiation long before you are subjected to that type of treatment, and I hope you never are. That preventive element is the one that distinguishes my approach to health problems.

Over the years I've been asked too many questions about therapy for which I am inclined to say, "You should have asked me twenty years ago." As the fabric of nutrition is examined and more of its threads are understood, there is more and more of an overall pattern to be discerned, and you can begin to fully use nutrition as I like to see it used: preventively.

2 | COMPLEX PROBLEMS OF ESTROGEN

I don't know how many times over the years I've collided with physicians over prescribing estrogen—for menstrual irregularity, menopausal symptoms, infertility, contraception. Many of the problems women suffer from are caused by estrogen stimulation. It is paradoxical that estrogen is routinely used to treat conditions caused by estrogen. (It is not the only case where this is done. Irradiation causes cancer, yet large doses of radiation are used to treat cancer.) I will never agree to a woman in my family being treated with estrogen for any reason. It causes at least eleven varieties of cancer in five varieties of animals. As higher doses of estrogen are used the risk of breast cancer goes up sharply and the chance of endometrial cancer goes up by a factor of twelve.

There is little doubt that long-term estrogen replacement therapy causes endometrial cancer. The medical people say endometrial cancer is easy to deal with; if you catch it early, it's no problem. So they continue to give estrogen replacement therapy to menopausal women, hoping to catch the endometrial cancer early (which they should, as the patient will need to visit the physician regularly) instead of treating the menopausal symptoms nutritionally, which

25

can be done, and eliminating the higher risk of developing the cancer.

There is some evidence that use of the pill lessens the chance of uterine cancer, and that protection lasts for five years after the pill is stopped. But there is also evidence that the hormones in the pill cause uterine cancer. My philosophy: When the scientists disagree, the only possible path for the public to choose is the one that is safest. Thousands of middle-aged women will develop cancer of the uterus from being given menopausal drugs containing estrogen they don't need. Of the 800,000 hysterectomies performed in this country in one year, one-third of them were unnecessary; one thousand of them were fatal.

In the 1950s a synthetic estrogen, diethylstilbestrol (DES), was prescribed for millions of women to prevent spontaneous abortion in pregnancy. DES was later found to cause cancer and precancerous conditions and uterine and testicular abnormalities in the offspring of the women who took it. And this was only a *synthetic* estrogen.

Many medical people argue that the case against estrogen as causing or promoting cancer has been largely disproved. Risk-benefit ratio is frequently used to justify estrogen hormone treatment for various disorders, including menopausal symptoms and osteoporosis. Another factor often cited as offsetting the risks of estrogen is a "better quality of life." In other words, a menopausal woman taking estrogen is not worried about fractures from a weakened skeleton caused by osteoporosis and is not upset by sweats and flushes and so has a better quality of life—and doesn't that offset the risks of estrogen? Yet research has shown that there is little doubt long-term estrogen therapy causes endometrial cancer, and that in high doses it also increases the risk of breast cancer.

You can protect the skeleton with adequate intake of cod-liver oil, which contains vitamins A and D and calcium. This needs to be done long before menopause: If you wait until then, that's crisis intervention. As for flushes, vitamin E, ginseng tea, and riboflavonoids will provide relief. The risk-benefit ratio doesn't exist in the nutritional approach because it's all benefit and no risk.

Many years ago I journeyed to Cincinnati to debate a premise to which I took violent exception: that the birth-control pill was safe. One of the palpable dangers is that the pill throws a woman into a state of simulated pregnancy for ten, twenty, thirty years, and no one can make a prediction of what happens when you create that simulated state. Beyond that there is a tacit admission of danger, since women are told that when they reduce the dose they reduce the danger. But if there wasn't any danger in the first place, why reduce the dose to lessen it in the second? A round-up of the hazards of the birth-control pill is largely a round-up of the hazards of estrogen.

Young women rested their hopes for safe contraception on the birth-control pill and learned they swallowed a lot more than a pill of estrogen and progesterone: They were at increased risk of blood clots, heart attack, and stroke. Studies now show long-term pill users have up to triple the risk of heart attack and the risk lasts for twenty years after the pills are no longer taken. If you smoke, heart attack risk increases, especially if you have taken the pill consistently for five or more years and are thirty-five or older. Blood clots—a key component in the risk of stroke and heart attack—remain a danger. The number of pill users at high risk is about 6 percent according to some estimates. If you have a history of breast cancer, you increase the risk if you take the pill or estrogen in any other form.

Estrogen also interacts with many drugs. You seldom leave a doctor's office without a prescription. It has often been cited as an example of male chauvinism that women tend to leave the doctor's office with a prescription for tranquilizers more frequently than men do. (A woman's symptoms are often blamed on "hysteria," which comes from the Greek word for uterus.) It was discovered that if a woman is taking the pill, Valium will not be broken down in the

27

body the way it normally is—the pill interferes with the breakdown.

When under the control of the hormones in the birth-control pill, a woman's body thinks it's pregnant, and this affects the amount of fluid in the cornea of the eye, just as in an actual pregnancy. Retention of fluid can thicken the cornea and so affects the type of contact lenses you can wear (those worn for extended periods can cause very severe problems). Most women wouldn't find this a problem for the nine months of a pregnancy, but it would be of great concern to many who are prescribed estrogen, whether in birth-control pills or for other conditions, for a period of several years.

In examining the medical histories of 1500 women, investigators at the University of North Carolina and Duke University Medical Center found that estrogen used to control menopausal symptoms increased the risk of breast cancer for women who underwent natural (rather than surgically produced) menopause by about 1.7 percent. But, there was no increased risk among women who had undergone hysterectomies. Women who received estrogen orally also had no significantly increased risk, but those who received estrogen by injection had a risk of developing breast cancer that was four times the norm. Why would estrogen taken orally have less risk than when taken by injection? Because the estrogen does not follow the same route in the body. When taken by injection, the estrogen bypasses the liver.

The hormone needs to be regulated, whether you are taking it by prescription or manufacturing it yourself, and it is regulated by the liver. The liver must deal with the hormone or you are in danger. Excessive intake of sugar and inadequate intake of protein and vitamin B complex will prevent the liver from doing its job. If you eat white bread, white sugar, and white rice, seldom eat organ meats, never use brewer's yeast, wheat germ, or desiccated liver, you are letting estrogen break away from its chains, removing it from control and asking for trouble. You can see when this is beginning to happen.

28

The early signs of trouble are premenstrual syndrome, fluid retention, backache, cramps, irritability, hysteria, dizziness, and cravings for sweets in the premenstrual week.

Next is a lengthening of the menstrual period. A five-day menstrual period is average, but if you use less sugar and eat adequate protein and increase your intake of vitamin B complex, the five-day period frequently becomes three days.

I'm convinced five days is average, but it's not normal. Furthermore, it is evidence of a process that can lead to estrogen-dependent cancer.

The third stage of estrogen-related difficulties reveals itself in cystic breast disease, endometriosis, uterine fibroids, or breast or uterine cancer.

Some medical people argue that if women are given progesterone along with estrogen, the progesterone protects them against the cancer-causing action of estrogen—yet many doctors still give estrogen by injection without the progesterone. But progesterone production is hastened and heightened by vitamin B_6. If indeed progesterone is an antidote for estrogen, which it may be, it can be safely stimulated by taking vitamin B_6 rather than by pills or injections. Vitamin B complex in the diet is a critical factor in controlling estrogen, whether it is prescribed by a doctor or produced by the ovaries.

Thirty-six years ago a Canadian study was done on a group of women with breast cancer. Two variables were studied: how much of the B vitamins they had in their systems and how much estrogen. The researcher had a suspicion that when you have low vitamin B and high estrogen you are a candidate for breast cancer. The study compared two groups of women, one group with breast cancer and one group without, for those two factors. In the group of women with breast cancer, 94.5 percent had high estrogen and low vitamin B, while 94.5 percent of the other group had high estrogen and higher vitamin B. Notice that the percentage was identical.

The significance of this is simple: B vitamins are needed to control

29

estrogen. The estrogen you yourself produce is just as much a threat as the estrogen prescribed for the menopause or in the birth-control pill. The evidence from this study implies that physicians should never prescribe the birth-control pill without raising the intake of vitamin B complex. In fact, it goes beyond that: You should also lower sugar intake and take precautions to see that protein intake is adequate.

Vitamin B complex cuts down excess activity of estrogen, whether prescribed for menopause or birth control or produced by the woman's own ovaries.

All too often physicians want to dose women with hormones to achieve a result that can be achieved totally harmlessly with a group of vitamins that have been removed from processed bread, rice, spaghetti, corn, buckwheat, and rye. It would be better for all of us if they tried instead to do something about the removal of these vitamins from foods; then we would not need to supplement our diets with B complex to put back what is removed from the majority of products sold in the supermarket.

The longer a woman is exposed to estrogen, the more at risk she is. Early menstruation and late menopause extend the period of risk. An eight-year study of two hundred school girls conducted at the University of Helsinki, Finland, found that those who had their first menstruation relatively young are at an increased risk of developing breast cancer in later life. Women who began to menstruate before the age of twelve are twice as likely to develop breast cancer as those who began at thirteen or later. Early menstruation obviously means several years of additional exposure to increased estrogen stimulation. There is the same risk to women who have a late menopause, for exactly the same reason.

During pregnancy estrogen levels go up, and yet pregnancy early in life, before the age of twenty-five, is protective against breast cancer. How can we explain that? Estrogen becomes safe when the body breaks it down into estriol, which is done in the liver. The

American Medical Association has stated that "the evidence that estriol is safe has piled so high that we should not be waiting for the last 'i' to be dotted." Yet doctors continue to prescribe estrogen and not the more-expensive-to-produce estriol. (I will never have enough financial backing to overcome the fact that the estrogen on the market, which comes from the urine of pregnant mares, is awfully cheap, and the companies producing it have a lot of money to spend on advertising and medical journals.)

In pregnancy the extra estrogen is broken down into estriol if the woman is properly nourished. In fact, if the estriol level is low in early pregnancy, there is the possibility of miscarriage. (This makes sense if you stop to think about it, since estrogen is used for birth control.) The breaking down of estrogen into estriol is therefore protective of the fetus.

The function in the body of breaking estrogen down into estriol, a hormone that presents no danger, is a diet-dependent function. It is disturbed by too much sugar, it is disturbed by too little protein, and it is incapacitated almost completely by lack of vitamin B complex.

It isn't only the estrogen that is prescribed at menopause or in birth-control pills that should concern you. The estrogen your own body produces has the same potential for mischief if either of two circumstances exist: your estrogen level is too high; or you don't break it down into estriol because of poor diet.

It has been reported that there is an estrogenic value in certain types of whiskey. This may explain why alcoholic males become impotent or sterile and some have enlargement of the breasts. The estrogenic value of whiskey may be a hazard to women, too. An alcoholic is someone who substitutes alcohol for food and is therefore nutritionally deficient. Liver damage from alcohol is proverbial—you've heard of cirrhosis of the liver. It is possible the impotence, sterility, and breast enlargement of the male alcoholic do not come from the estrogen in the whiskey or from that estrogen alone. The

31

liver breaks down estrogen; when the liver is sick it doesn't do it. And the liver is slow to respond to an improved diet, even when it is badly needed.

Control of estrogen activity in the body rests in part on the capacity of the liver to break down the hormone, which in turn depends on adequate dietary supplies of vitamin B complex, particularly choline and inositol. Adequate protein is also needed to help the liver break down estrogenic hormone. This is the chemistry that will help a woman to mitigate, if not avoid, such disorders as cystic mastitis, endometriosis, uterine fibroid tumors, and breast cancer. One woman in eleven is a target for breast cancer. I'm not talking about an academic subject.

Control of estrogen is a *nutritional* process; it is not properly achieved by prescribing more estrogen.

Medical people seem to feel estrogen is not important before you get cancer, and only then do they try to control it—with drug therapy. But women need not suffer unnecessarily with premenstrual tension, backache, cramps, water retention, drawing pain, sensitive breasts, longer periods and hemorrhaging; or develop cystic mastitis, which can be precancerous but can be mitigated and even prevented; or have hysterectomies for uterine fibroids that can shrink through proper nutrition; or be subjected to surgery for endometriosis, which can be controlled nutritionally.

A woman needs to control estrogen *before* she becomes concerned about premenstrual syndrome or a prolonged period or cystic mastitis or fibroid tumors. She can shrink the fibroids, reverse the endometriosis, control or eliminate premenstrual problems. My thesis is that she may then be preventing estrogen-dependent cancer.

To focus attention on the estrogen produced by a cow and passed along in cheese is to forget that every woman produces estrogen. If it's dangerous in the cheese, what is it when it comes from her own ovaries?

The body has a built-in regulating mechanism to control estrogen: the liver. But that mechanism is diet-dependent. If you don't eat properly it won't work. Fat is not the culprit—I have actually used high-fat diets to bring estrogenic hormone activity down. It isn't fat and it isn't red meat that are wreaking havoc on the liver: It is sugar and caffeine and buying foods deprived of vitamin B complex, which is essential to the hormone-regulating mechanism of the body. Without that regulation estrogen intermittently stimulates the breast and uterus—and intermittent stimulation is often worse than steady stimulation; the body would develop a mechanism for dealing with something steady. The controlling mechanism based on vitamin B complex is supported by adequate protein. It is impaired or destroyed by too much sugar; caffeine does not help it and may indeed hurt it.

There is a direct link between sugar intake and breast cancer in older women. In a research study of sugar consumption and breast cancer in twenty-one countries, no type of sweetener gave a better correlation than total sucrose, although some data on glucose consumption tended to implicate it more strongly than sucrose. The medical establishment has only recently acknowledged that sugar consumption is more closely related to breast-cancer mortality than is fat consumption. And it appears that diet plays a far more important role in fatal breast cancer in older women than in younger ones. Insulin is the link between sugar intake and breast cancer; diabetics are at increased risk for breast cancer. For insulin levels to remain within normal range, the first step is to get rid of sugar. If you were able to cut out all the sugar in your diet—which is impossible—you would lose thirty-four pounds in twelve months. Excessive consumption of sugar leads to obesity, and obesity is linked very definitely with breast cancer.

For alleviating menopausal symptoms there are many natural nutritional means that can bring relief from sweats and flushes— ginseng tea, vitamin E, bioflavonoids. Atrophic vaginitis can be treated with a combination of vitamin A cream and vitamin E cream. This is a successful substitute for an estrogen cream. (A dose of estrogen in a vaginal cream, which is absorbed into the body, is

33

exactly equivalent to a dose of estrogen by mouth.) For cystic breast disease, choline, inositol, lecithin, vitamin E, a caffeine-free diet, reduced sugar intake, and increased protein take care of the problem without the need for an estrogen prescription. For premenstrual syndrome vitamin B complex and vitamin B$_6$ are most helpful; the medical establishment's tendency to treat PMS with estrogen or birth-control pills (which combine estrogen and progesterone) brings the potential for iatrogenic disease—disease induced by a doctor.

We are told by doctors that if you give progesterone with estrogen it acts as a safe counterbalance. The American woman follows a diet low in vitamin B$_6$ and her progesterone production is therefore inadequate without it. That is why progesterone produced in the body does not protect that one woman in eleven who is getting breast cancer. As one commentator said, "If breast cancer were a male disease a national emergency would be declared by the chauvinistic male medical establishment."

Doctors say as women go into menopause their estrogen level goes down and this causes sweats and flushes. If so, why don't ten-year-old girls, who are low in estrogen, have sweats and flushes? Why don't men have them? In the one double-blind, carefully controlled study of the effectiveness of estrogen measured against a placebo in controlling menopausal sweats and flushes, the placebo more effectively controlled the symptoms than the estrogen did.

What can be done nutritionally when, for some compelling reason, a physician insists a woman is sorely in need of estrogen? Sugar and caffeine should be removed from the diet; intake of vitamin B complex, especially choline and inositol, should be raised to help the body control estrogen the way it is supposed to be controlled— by the liver. And there are additional benefits: Uterine tumors sometimes shrink, endometriosis sometimes responds, premenstrual symptoms sometimes vanish or are alleviated. More important, the body has been equipped to deal with estrogen the way it is supposed to.

3 | ESTROGEN-STIMULATED DISORDERS

Menstrual Irregularities

In the 1940s, Dr. Morton Briskind (whom I worked with when I was director of the education department of a large vitamin laboratory headed by Dr. Casimir Funk, the man who isolated vitamin B_1 in 1912 and who originated the word vitamin) published a paper entitled "Nutritional Therapy of Endocrine Disturbances" in which he described the effect of vitamin B complex in reducing the length of time of a woman's menstrual flow from five or six days to three or four days. He found that patients with mild to moderate signs of B complex deficiency that appeared during the week before menstruation—increased nervous tension, insomnia, tenderness of the breasts, a feeling of fullness, stuffiness, lumbar backache, headache, fatigue, low abdominal cramps—reported that menstruation came on "completely without warning" while they were on vitamin B complex therapy. He was describing premenstrual syndrome, PMS, which only recently has been recognized by the medical establishment as a disease. And he treated it successfully through nutrition, not drugs.

On the other hand, Briskind found that women with signs of more serious and protracted B complex deficiency, who suffered from exaggerated menstrual hemorrhaging, reported more severe pain when vitamin B complex therapy was begun. However, in virtually every case where this occurred, there was little or no pain during subsequent periods while the nutritional therapy was continued. That is, in women with severe premenstrual syndrome the symptoms were worse in the first month after vitamin B complex therapy was begun, but were greatly relieved as therapy continued.

This happens because the vitamin initially increases hormone activity, and most of these problems are caused by estrogenic hormone. The liver, which is the target for the vitamin B complex therapy, takes a long time to respond, and until it does the estrogen activity is not yet brought under control. It usually takes less than a month for hormone activity to go up in response to improved nutrition, but it takes two months for the liver to respond. Therefore estrogen-related menstrual problems—premenstrual syndrome, severe hemorrhaging, excessively long menstrual periods, endometriosis—as well as other estrogen-related diseases, such as cystic mastitis and fibroid tumors, may become worse in the first month of nutritional treatment; it is not until the second month that the therapeutic benefit begins.

Large doses of estrogen are often prescribed for these conditions. Because the estrogen depresses the menstrual cycle, it seems as though it has a therapeutic effect. When prescribed for excessive hemorrhaging during the menstrual period, estrogen will suppress the normal cycle and there will be little or no bleeding. However, estrogen prescribed this way does not identify or correct the underlying problem, and may actually make it worse.

The process that causes premenstrual syndrome, the same process that makes the average American woman's menstruation time abnormal—which she doesn't realize because many share this abnormal pattern—is one that can easily come under dietary control.

For many years it was fashionable for the medical profession to be indifferent to nutrition. Over those years I learned that nutritional approaches can be used for reducing premenstrual syndrome, for shortening the overlong menstrual period, for control of excessive hemorrhaging, and, in some cases, for endometriosis, as well as for shrinking or dissolving breast cysts and halting the growth of uterine fibroids or even shrinking them.

You hear vitamin B_6 spoken of as though it were the one single answer to the problems of premenstrual syndrome. I'm not only talking about problems during the premenstrual week; I'm also talking about a menstrual period that is longer than three or, at most, four days. The reason five or six or seven days is considered normal is that so many women endure that. In those years of close observation, working with physicians, I developed a formulation which was able to do the following (not in all cases; there are no panaceas): shorten the menstrual period from an average of five days to an average of three days; reduce premenstrual symptoms; shrink, or even totally dissolve, the cysts of cystic breast disease; halt the growth of, or even shrink, uterine fibroid tumors.

The diet has to be low in sugar; caffeine must be eliminated; food allergies must be eliminated. The diet must be high in protein.

Vitamin B complex formulated with adequate quantities of the factors involved in fat metabolism (estrogen is fat soluble) is needed. These are the lipotropic factors, and include choline and inositol. They are also antioxidants that provide protection against cancer and act as antiaging factors.

The chemistry involved here in shortening the menstrual period also helps to protect against endometriosis, uterine fibroid tumors, cystic breast disease, and estrogen-dependent breast cancer.

When you give vitamin B_6 to women in the premenstrual week or start a little earlier, at ovulation, there is an enormously beneficial effect on such symptoms as fluid retention, cramps, and anxiety. In short, you normalize the menstrual process. These women would

37

not show a response if they did not need the vitamin to begin with. I want you to consider one other thing: Every woman who is on the pill has a vitamin B_6 deficiency because the pill causes it.

Irregular Periods and Amenorrhea

Irregular periods and amenorrhea (lack of menstruation) can be caused by excess body fat (being overweight can actually interfere with the entire reproductive system). The fat has the capacity for elaborating hormones, and the hormone load that is elaborated disturbs the balances in the body. A sensible diet and gradual weight loss will usually serve to regularize the menstrual cycle once you reach your normal weight.

When there has been amenorrhea, PABA and folic acid treatments have sometimes been successful. There is some evidence that the ovaries can be stimulated nutritionally. Even in cases where there is a hereditary defect, often some type of enzyme deficiency, it may be possible to improve the condition nutritionally. Sometimes the enzyme, if there's any of it at all, can be stimulated. The building blocks for enzymes, among other things, in addition to protein, frequently include vitamins and sometimes minerals, depending on whether you are talking about an enzyme or an apoenzyme.

Some years ago an endocrinologist in Boston was working with a group of women who, for a period of five years, had been unable to conceive. Through treatment with a single nutrient, paraaminobenzoic acid, he harvested a crop of twelve babies in the twenty-two women in two years! This indicates that a profound effect on the reproductive tract probably mediates via the pituitary. It is for this reason I caution women high in estrogen—women subject to cystic breast disease—regarding the use of PABA and folic acid. I don't mind a small quantity, but I have seen some cases of cystic mastitis worsen from doses of PABA and folic acid.

There was a report on young chickens dosed with paraaminobenzoic acid or folic acid: The result was an increase in the size of the oviduct—the egg-laying tube, which I guess would correspond roughly to the uterus in women. The increase was forty-fold. If a chick deficient in PABA or folic acid was given estrogen, the effect on the ovaries was minimal—only one-fourth of what it was when estrogen was given simultaneously with folic acid and PABA.

Premenstrual Syndrome. Premenstrual syndrome affects 80 percent of the women in this country to some degree, and 20 percent of them are generally incapacitated for one or more days a month. PMS is considered normal. But I've always felt a condition that makes a woman incapable of intellectual performance at her normal level one, two, three, or more days a month is not normal.

I'm gratified the medical establishment has decided to elevate premenstrual syndrome to the status of a disease, which means they now find it appropriate to treat it. (In England a few years ago there was a murder trial in which a woman who killed her husband was found not guilty on the grounds she was temporarily incompetent because of premenstrual syndrome.) Unfortunately, many orthodox physicians want to treat it with estrogen or birth-control pills when there exist successful nutritional treatments.

Women with signs of severe vitamin B complex deficiency reported dysmenorrhea or more severe pain at the start of vitamin B complex therapy; as the nutritional therapy continued, there was little or no pain. That is, in women with severe PMS the symptoms were worse in the first month after vitamin B complex therapy was begun, but in the following months the symptoms were greatly relieved.

Vitamin B complex cuts down excess activity of estrogen. Premenstrual syndrome is estrogen related and vitamin B complex initially increases hormone activity. The liver, which is the target for the B complex therapy, takes longer to respond, and until it does the estrogen is not under control. It usually takes less than a month for hormone activity to go up but two months for the liver to respond.

So the advice on treating PMS with estrogen or birth-control pills (which contain estrogen and progesterone) has created the potential for iatrogenic disease.

A recent review of premenstrual syndrome neatly summarized the benefits of improved nutrition for women who suffer that condition: Tension, anxiety, bloating, and weight gain are improved with two hundred to eight hundred milligrams of vitamin B_6 daily. Some patients benefit by eating less refined sugar (I would say most do), dairy products, animal fats, and using less caffeine and salt. Those who suffer from headache and dizziness and craving for sweets may be helped by linoleic acid, which is available in vegetable oils, plus increased intake of magnesium, zinc, niacinamide, and vitamin C. Women should also cut down on alcohol. Women suffering premenstrually from depression and insomnia, which goes hand in hand with depression, may owe their problems to something they don't suspect: elevated lead in the body. This too can be treated nutritionally. They may also have tyrosine deficiency. That's a protein acid—an amino acid—and supplements of this may be helpful.

Some women with amalgam fillings in their mouths may have mercury toxicity contributing to their troubles with premenstrual syndrome. That can only be established by a dentist who knows the subject and knows how to test for mercury poisoning, which is not simple (see chapter 5).

Women who have elevated blood copper are likely to become depressed, and histadine (an amino acid) is one of the treatments for depression induced by elevated blood copper.

Women sometimes have elevated blood copper in the week before menstruation, and this may be responsible for the depression some suffer at that time—brushed off by a male medical establishment as one of the prices for being female—but which turns out to be treatable.

Magnesium therapy to correct magnesium deficiency has been found helpful in women with premenstrual syndrome. I use vitamin B complex with large amounts of choline and inositol in helping relieve premenstrual syndrome symptoms. For some of these conditions you end up with a tranquilizer in an orthodox medical office. In the nutritionist's office, we make an attempt to correct the chemistry.

Diuretics, for those with a tendency to store water, are used to treat symptoms; they do not address the causes of water retention. Women who take diuretics need supplements because as they excrete water they are excreting other things as well.

Many women—I'd say most—with premenstrual syndrome, particularly when bloating and sensitivity of the breasts are present, benefit by supplements of vitamin B complex. The type of vitamin B complex used is important. The manufacturers tend to give you an impressive list of individual B vitamins with a generous amount of B_1 and B_2 and niacin. When they get to choline and inositol, they either don't put them in or the amount that is put in seems to make the label impressive but serves no useful purpose. It's too low. I find that a worthwhile vitamin B complex supplement should supply one thousand milligrams of choline and five hundred milligrams of inositol in the recommended supplementary intake. I often combine that with evening primrose oil and some of the nutrients I listed earlier.

Vitamin E is helpful in premenstrual syndrome when PMS is accompanied by cystic breast disease without malignancy. The next time you run into a physician who is a skeptic about the use of vitamin E for premenstrual syndrome, you might point out that the information on vitamin E came from an article in the *Journal of the American Medical Association*, which the orthodox physician is likely to regard with some awe if not trepidation. Vitamin E in the form of dl-alpha tocopheral was given in doses of 150, 300, or 600 units daily. There was significant improvement in control of nervous tension, mood swings, irritability, anxiety, headache, craving for

41

sweets, increased appetite, pounding of the heart, fatigue, dizziness, fainting, depression, forgetfulness, crying, confusion, and insomnia. There were no significant changes in weight gain with vitamin E, or swelling of the extremities, breast tenderness, and abdominal bloating. This was a controlled study in which some women took a placebo—something that looked like a vitamin E capsule but actually was inactive. That's to get rid of the power of suggestion. No symptoms of toxicity were experienced. The optimal dose of vitamin E, the researchers concluded, was 300 units daily.

Now, let me make two exceptions from my much larger experience with vitamin E than was enjoyed by the authors of that article. First, dl-alpha tocopheral is synthetic; it has less potency than natural vitamin E. Second, other forms of vitamin E are also valuable, especially for their antiaging effect. So, I prefer to recommend the mixed tocopherals of natural origin over the synthetic dl-alpha tocopheral, but even with that I'm still glad to see that in the medical literature—which for a long time assured us that vitamin E is a vitamin in search of a disease, that deficiency in vitamin E does not exist—we are at last getting recognition of what we in nutrition have known for almost half a century: It's a very valuable vitamin for some purposes, and premenstrual syndrome is one of them.

Evening primrose oil helps the body to manufacture prostaglandin E_1. The use of that oil in the treatment of premenstrual syndrome is a classic example of the difference between traditional medicine and medicine of the orthomolecular group. Typically, the traditional approach to premenstrual syndrome has been to prescribe painkillers, or analgesics; anti-inflammatory drugs, which reduce inflammation at a particular site; and hormones, particularly progesterone.

In my estimation, none of these approaches to PMS address the problem of what is going on biochemically at a cellular level. My recommendation is to take two capsules of English evening primrose oil about twenty minutes before meals three times a day, beginning two weeks before the menstrual period is due, and to continue this every day for three months. This is followed by a maintenance dose of one capsule three times a day.

When you give vitamin B_6 to menstruating women in the pre-menstrual week, or start a little earlier at ovulation, there is an enormously beneficial effect on such symptoms as fluid collection and water retention; there are fewer cramps, less anxiety. In short, you normalize the process. Women would not show that response if they did not need the vitamin B_6 to begin with. An index of deficiency in vitamin B_6 is to be seen by noting the French bread and the salty snacks and the white bread and the cake flour in the diets of PMS sufferers.

I want you to consider one other thing: Every woman who is on the pill has a vitamin B_6 deficiency because the pill causes it. Vitamin B_6 has become very important in offsetting some adverse effects of the birth-control pill. The oral contraceptives very often cause derangement of vitamin metabolism and as a result of this, there may be psychological disturbances. According to some reports, as many as 34 percent of users of the pill show mild to moderate depression and irritability, emotionalism, lethargy, and constant tiredness. Some of them even develop paranoid ideas. It turns out that an adverse effect on vitamin B_6 metabolism is involved, and investigators have been reporting that in as many as three women out of four with psychological upsets associated with the pill, fifty milligrams of vitamin B_6 daily produced marked improvement. Vitamin B_6 has also been helpful for women in offsetting the tendency to store water, particularly in the premenstrual week.

Most applications of B_6 to problems associated with the premenstrual week I have mentioned, but there is one more. Many women suffer outbreaks of acne just before their periods. In 72 percent of those taking 50 milligrams of the vitamin daily for one week before and during their period, these premenstrual flare-ups were relieved.

It is a problem deciding how much vitamin B_6 people need. Two milligrams is the recommended dietary allowance set by the medical establishment. That is simply erroneous for a large percentage of the population. In general, you can say that many people need 50 percent more than the RDA and some people need up to one thousand milligrams each day. That is unusual, but it does occur; there are schizophrenics who need that much.

Vitamin B$_6$ is widely distributed in foods. It is found in beef liver, kidney, pork loin, ham, veal, fresh fish, bananas, cabbage, avocados, peanuts, walnuts, raisins, prunes, and cereal grains. But the losses in processing are great. Vegetables lose some of their vitamin B$_6$ in freezing, and in canning high temperatures are used for safety and for sterilization, and this too destroys the vitamin. Some provision has been made for enrichment of flour and bread with vitamin B$_6$ but no attention is paid to it. Vitamin B$_6$ and pantothenic acid and vitamin E are still discarded during milling and are still not restored.

Premenstrual syndrome and multiple allergies are two problems associated with yeast infections, but that link is not often made by the public. Many women develop premenstrual syndrome as a result of hormone dysfunction triggered by *Candida albicans*. (See chapter 5.)

Endometriosis

Uncontrolled levels of estrogen have been indicted for contributing to the serious problem of endometriosis. The process that leads to endometriosis, and to cystic breast disease and uterine fibroid tumors, can be, in part, the process that leads to breast cancer.

Some cases of endometriosis have responded to nutritional therapy and some have not. A medical nutritionist can approach this problem by suggesting the type of nutrition that will bring the estrogen level down in the normal way: increasing vitamin B$_6$ intake and protein consumption and decreasing sugar and caffeine in the diet. This will encourage the liver to control the estrogen, which in many women isn't doing its job because of their poor diet.

Physicians often suggest oral contraceptives to treat severe endometriosis. This is an attempt to use the antidotal properties of progesterone, which is an ingredient in most (but not all) birth-control pills. But use of birth-control pills for the benefit of the progesterone contained in them is often not necessary, since progesterone can be stimulated nutritionally with vitamin B_6.

Cystic Breast Disease

There are instances where I feel women have been subjected to surgery that conceivably could be avoided, where they have been given symptomatic treatment rather than therapy aimed at the cause of the problem and where they have been subjected to hazards, some of which have not been properly defined. One of these involves fibrocystic disease.

Cystic mastitis has been listed as a risk factor for breast cancer, although not a very strong one—not all women, nor even a sizable percentage of women, with cystic mastitis go on to develop the more serious disease. On the other hand, there is a movement in medicine to stop labeling cystic mastitis as a disease, and the reasoning behind this fascinates but infuriates me: So many people have it, it's normal.

I've had a great deal of experience in the nutritional management of cystic mastitis, and I don't want women to surrender to surgery for this condition because surgery attacks the symptom—the cyst—and not the cause.

A letter I received from Zion, Illinois, reads:

Dear Dr. Fredericks,
    I think it is important for all of us to get feedback in

45

everything we do, and I wanted to tell you of the spec-
tacular results I obtained after following your advice concerning fibrocystic disease. I followed your program . . .
with the cooperation of my doctor. Currently, I am free
from pain entirely, and my breast tissue has once again
become soft.

The onset of this ordeal began a year ago. I experienced
terrible pain from ovulation until the seventh or eighth
day of the cycle, so you can see there weren't too many
good days left, and my gynecologist said there was nothing
I could do. Only after I developed three large cysts did
the medical practitioners feel they could intervene. I went
to see two surgeons, and in the end the result was that I
did have out-patient surgery to remove the cysts.

Let me note that that is symptomatic treatment, and every physician is taught that symptomatic treatment is a compromise that
you adopt only reluctantly.

However, as you mention, medicine can only treat the
end product. I had almost instant results from the inclu-
sion in my diet of more vitamin E and vitamin B_6. The
initial results waned somewhat. I would say the total re-
covery took about six months. Abandoning caffeine and
chocolate, to which I was addicted, has helped enormously, and the estrogen levels really seem to be under
control with the addition of choline and inositol; and my
periods have become shorter and lighter as a result of the
lowering of the estrogen. I cannot begin to thank you
enough for your assessment of this problem. You are right
on target. I have shared this near miracle with all my
friends, and they have been helped too. Your name is a
household word in my neighborhood. Thank you again
ever so much.

In a study on the relationship between caffeine and cystic breast disease, daily caffeine consumption from coffee, tea, cola, and chocolate was estimated in 634 women with fibrocystic disease and 1,000 women with unrelated conditions. A significantly greater risk of fibrocystic disease was seen with increasing caffeine intake. The women who took the equivalent of five to six cups of coffee a day (meaning they could have been taking tea or cola or chocolate in equal amounts to that of caffeine in coffee) were 2.3 times as likely to have fibrocystic breast disease as those who took the equivalent of a single cup. The relative risk was especially high for certain specialized types of fibrocystic breast disease; no elevated risk was found for benign breast disease.

Premenstrual breast symptoms were positively associated with the use of caffeine by the controls but not in the other cases, showing that the body of a woman may react in one of two ways (but not both) to an excessive use of caffeine. In one group there are disturbances in the premenstrual week and in the second group the disturbance is centered in the breasts. That is something you ought to realize when you consider the impact of the endless advertising for caffeine-containing soft drinks and beverages in the media.

The letter I received from the woman in Illinois was very exciting and gratifying. It is my hope that in bringing estrogen under control through this nutritional approach and alleviating premenstrual syndrome, cystic breast disease, and uterine fibroid tumors, we may have an influence on the dreadful statistics which now say that one in eleven women will have breast cancer, and that one-third of all breast cancers are estrogen-dependent.

Another woman wrote me:

> I am a victim of cystic mastitis (fibrocystic disease). I'm in my early forties and I have had it since age twenty-five. I've been operated on three times because it forms up as tumors and the surgeon tells me if he doesn't take them out, he can't positively tell me what they are. Thank

God, all three times they have been benign. I asked him
about vitamin E. He said to take four hundred international units a day, two hundred IUs at a time, and in
addition take vitamin B complex with vitamin C three
times a day (at 11:00 A.M., 3:00 P.M., and at bedtime)
between meals. If I take them with food or if I have eaten,
have I negated the value of the vitamin and why has he
told me this? So long as I am getting the vitamins down
am I getting the value out of them?

When you eat a slice of whole wheat bread containing vitamin
B complex, does the fact that you are taking that vitamin with food
cancel the vitamin's effect? No! Vitamins belong with food. This
is like asking whether you should use spark plugs with gasoline.
The doctor was making an attempt to get a hormone (estrogen)
under control and doing it very well, but that hormone is fat soluble
and therefore the vitamins that affect fats—inositol and choline—
become critical. In the average vitamin B complex preparation,
these particular vitamins are usually either not present or they are
present in only token quantities.

One doctor who picked up on my work wrote an article entitled
"A Case of Cystic Mastitis." In the article he acknowledged two
approaches: "My patients and I are grateful to Dr. John A. Myers
of Baltimore and Dr. Carlton Fredericks for pioneering work in the
area of women's health problems leading to the solution which is
presented in this paper. The remedy described is an adaptation and
combination of the work of two men."

The doctor tells the story of a patient who came to his office
with cystic mastitis, saying:

One doctor said I should have my breasts removed
because I might get cancer. Another one said I did find
myself at more risk of cancer, but it wasn't all that much
more, so maybe I should wait and see. My regular doctor

48

agreed with that and said I should have mammography of the breasts every six months to identify any problem early because identifying it early is protective, and then have surgery if I need it. I have had a lot of X ray in my lifetime and I'm worried because X rays can cause cancer, too. The doctors tell me that I have fibrocystic disease— one doctor said "cystic mastitis" but that is the same thing, isn't it? I have had it badly about seven or eight years but, actually, I have had trouble with my breasts all my adult life. When I was in my twenties I would get tenderness, and also as a teenager. I get tenderness just before the menstrual period and again the doctors disagree. Some tell me it is normal; some tell me it is not.

Well, this particular doctor said it is not normal; it is not even necessary. He said it is a commentary on the nutritional status of women that an abnormality is counted as being normal. As I read that note I was reminded of a doctor (and I hope he is retired now, really) who said he examined women for hypoglycemia (low blood sugar) and he found so many cases he decided hypoglycemia is normal. So, if you have false teeth, that is normal because a lot of other people have false teeth. This woman said exactly what I've heard so often before:

For nearly twenty years I've had to wear a bra to bed. At first, it was mostly before the menstrual period. Then, in my early thirties I began to get some cysts, and when they appeared I was scared to death. I thought it was cancer. My doctor said, "Just fibrocystic disease. A lot of women have it; don't worry about it." But when I started getting more lumps and pain was not confined to the premenstrual week but all the time, I was so bad before the menstrual period that my doctor gave me diuretics to drain the fluid. I found they helped a little but they didn't

49

really do the job and I didn't like using a drug. After I turned forty, I had two lumps which were so painful and so large I had to have them drained with needles.

Incidentally, that woman's concern about diuretics is intelligent. When diuretics take water out of the body, they also take out nutrients. Unfortunately, that wasn't recognized for a long time. When they became aware that people were dropping on the street with potassium deficiency, they started to put potassium back. But they still haven't put back the other nutrients like zinc, for instance, which the diuretics remove.

This is all symptomatic treatment: draining the cysts with a needle, removing them surgically. This is treating the end of the process. There isn't a medical school in the whole world that doesn't teach medical students that symptomatic treatment is not the way to go because you are temporizing with the problem; you are not reaching the core.

She continues:

> Sometimes I can hardly bear to touch myself. My mother had the same problem, and after she was in menopause it seemed to die down a bit, but then she had to have a breast removed for cancer. And that is when the surgeon told me I should do the same thing: I should have my breasts removed to prevent cancer.
>
> When the surgeon told me I should have my breasts removed to prevent cancer, that's when I decided to look for alternatives. To me that seemed like committing suicide to prevent old age.

Here, I am stopping again to say that the removal of normal breasts on the basis of cysts represents a type of medicine to which I would never refer a woman and, certainly, would not permit any woman in my family to patronize. I have been very much shocked by the fact that there are girls as young as fourteen who have been subjected to this type of surgery, bilateral mastectomy, with the breasts normal, with no cancer. It is called prevention. In two of those cases I looked up the risk factors which the doctor listed as the reason for doing this surgery, and their interpretation was completely awry. I took those factors to a geneticist, somebody who knows how to evaluate risk factors, and the comment was, "The operation should never have been performed." What I am saying is, it is awfully good to get a second opinion from somebody who doesn't do surgery when that kind of a recommendation is made.

In this case, the doctor didn't go along with the recommendation for surgery. He examined the patient and found numerous lumps— large ones, small ones, hard ones, soft ones, the left side worse than the right but both of them bad. He told the patient it was too bad she couldn't have done something about this ten years before because it was a severe case but not to be discouraged because, even in severe cases, treatment usually brings substantial relief. He added that treatment is not drugs; it is *nutritional*. Although part of it may look like the application of a drug, actually the entire therapy is nutritional.

The doctor explained to the patient:

> I have learned how to treat this from a wise old doctor in Baltimore, Maryland, who had been doing clinical research with minerals for years. In less severe cases, diets properly arranged and oral supplementation are frequently sufficient. In your case, the method recommended by Dr. Myers should be followed. This emphasizes iodine and magnesium and sometimes they have to be given in a special way. The iodine is painted on extravaginally and the magnesium is injected intravenously immediately after the iodine is put on, and that is done sometimes once a week, sometimes more often. In addition to that, there are changes in diet: no refined sugar, no white bread, no

51

refined flour products. Make your diet as fresh as possible, use frozen foods rather than canned or packaged, eliminate artificial flavors, colors, and preservatives.

There are no guarantees in medicine, there never are, but this system works very well.

When she came back he asked her how she made out. She told him that when she got that injection, she felt warm all over, particularly in the pelvic area and throat. (This is usual.) The doctor asked if she had started changing her diet. She said, "Yes, and my husband is complaining."

The doctor then gave her a list of supplements to take:

- Vitamin B_6, one hundred milligrams three times daily. This helps the production of prolactin, a hormone that is frequently out of proportion in women with premenstrual syndrome. It also helps to counteract the effects of high levels of estrogen which has not been detoxified by the liver.
- Vitamin B complex, which backs up the high dose of vitamin B_6.
- Iodine. Kelp is not enough in as severe a case as this woman suffered from. (A prescription is needed for a higher potency than is available in the form of kelp.) The iodine also helps to reduce the production of estrogen.
- Magnesium, because magnesium and vitamin B_6 work together.
- A polyunsaturated fatty acid in capsule form (I actually prefer it on salad), which makes the iodine more available.
- Vitamin E. (Twenty years ago I was telling the public that vitamin E helps to prevent or reverse cystic mastitis and it wasn't until 1981 that the *Journal of the American Medical Association* announced it as a brand-new discovery. Isn't it nice they caught up?)

The thyroid hormone and estrogen hormone are antagonistic. If the estrogen goes up—which happens when women don't have enough of the B vitamins and protein and have too much sugar—the thyroid hormone goes down. Then, in addition to premenstrual syndrome, the woman may end up with dry skin, constipation, colds, and fatigue; she may feel chilled when other people are not and need more clothing than other people, considering the temperature. These are all profound reactions for a small change in the endocrine system in the glandular balances in the body. There is one other point: High or normal thyroid hormone is protective against cancer; low thyroid hormone invites it. High estrogen invites cancer; normal estrogen discourages it.

The woman was examined after a period of time. Many of the cystic lumps were slightly smaller. There was still tenderness but it took more pressure to elicit the tenderness, and the doctor recommended that she continue the treatment. The woman herself said the pain was much less and she could tell something was working. Because she had a very severe case, it took eight months before her fibrocystic problem was resolved. Her breasts became soft and pain-free. She didn't have to wear a bra to bed anymore. And she had no further premenstrual problems. The doctor concludes his report with a list of recommended reading, including one of my books on this subject. Control of estrogen is a nutritional process. The doctor took advantage of that knowledge. May his tribe be legion!

Uterine Fibroid Tumors

The very same nutritional therapy used to control fibrocystic disease has been used effectively to shrink uterine fibroid tumors in many cases. Often, fibroid tumors are stimulated by estrogen and therefore can be brought under control when estrogen production in the body is brought under control.

53

I ran into much professional indifference on this subject during the years when it was fashionable for professionals to be indifferent to nutritionists. One gynecologist called me because his patient insisted that she might be able to escape a hysterectomy for uterine fibroids with a nutritional approach. His mind was open and I gave him the details, a protocol, of the approach and he applied it. The fibroids did shrink (they don't in every case) and the hysterectomy was avoided. I referred another woman with fibroid tumors to that same gynecologist and he didn't apply the nutritional therapy; he went ahead and did a hysterectomy. A few days later I told this to one of his colleagues who knew about the first case and asked him why he didn't try the nutritional therapy. "Did he fall back into a habit?" His colleague said, "No. You can charge $75 or $100 for a consultation on a nutritional matter. You can charge $1500 or $2000 for surgery." I hope that was not the reason.

In another case a woman who developed cystic mastitis along with uterine fibroid tumors was treated at the medical center: Thirty-two years old, she was faced with a hysterectomy. Because the cystic mastitis had been going on for a number of years, her physician was suggesting a mastectomy—he said it was better to have breast removal for a benign disease than to run the risk of breast cancer. Well, one can quarrel with that or agree with it, but there *is* something else that can be done when a woman has a disorder that may be triggered by estrogen (she had been taking estrogen in the form of birth-control pills, a factor that is frequently overlooked, and also had a high level of internally produced estrogen). Nutritional therapy for reducing the activity of estrogen is nothing bizarre. It uses the normal mechanism in the body for controlling a mischief-making hormone.

In this particular case, the woman's mastitis did not disappear entirely but became less troublesome. The interesting thing is what happened with her uterine fibroids. She went back to her doctor, who had consented grudgingly to nutritional therapy, telling her he didn't want to wait too long for the surgery because the fibroids were large. His examination found the tumors had been reduced from something the size of an orange to the size of a rosebud. She did not have the surgery!

I don't know entirely with how many cases of uterine fibroids we've been successful, but over the years I know of several dozen where nutritional therapy—high protein, low sugar, and increased intake of choline and inositol through supplements—has brought a shrinkage of uterine fibroids to the point where hysterectomies were avoided, sometimes in very young women, twenty-five or thirty years of age.

The protocol is not a panacea—it does not work for everybody. In some postmenopausal women, we have not been able to shrink the fibroids; if the woman is still not menopausal, we have a chance. The therapy is predicated on a nutritional method of removing from the fibroids the stimulation of estrogenic hormone activity.

4 | CANCER

Antioxidants

One of the reasons for retention of the characteristics of youth long after it has disappeared is a good intake of antioxidants. If I told a group of college graduates that there are factors in nutrition that prevent oxygen from attacking your cells, and if you prevent that you may prevent cancer and you may retard aging, do you think I'd make any headway? Don't be foolish. I've tried it. Well, the American Cancer Institute finally put up millions of dollars to study that which they fairly recently called quackery—the relationship of nutrition to both the prevention and treatment of cancer. The oxygen you breathe, which supports the flame of life, 98 percent of the time does just what it is supposed to do. The other 2 percent of the oxygen you breathe is a mischief-maker; it is altered by the chemistry of the body and becomes activated. The body's defense against this activity is waged by a number of nutrients and metabolites. These are called antioxidants because they block the excessive effects of activated oxygen. Nutrients come from the diet;

metabolites are manufactured within the body, usually from nutrients or break-down products.

One effect of activated oxygen in the body is to partially break or split molecules of compounds normal to the body. The abnormal molecules that are formed are electrically unbalanced and so will latch onto some other molecules, possibly in a place they do not belong. They are conducive to aging and are part of the aging process.

I'm not going into an elaborate explanation of antioxidants; I will start by simply saying that the side effects of irradiation include activated oxygen, which then causes chemical changes—free radical activity—which make for other reactions.

The working hypothesis suggests that free radicals, which are scavenged by antioxidants (such as vitamin C and vitamin E), are potentially carcinogenic. How does that work? Oxygen is needed by the body and one thinks of oxygen as indispensable and always desirable. But if you think of painters constantly painting steel bridges to keep them from rusting as a result of oxidation, you suddenly realize that oxygen can be an enemy.

Oxidation also occurs in human cells. It occurs in human cells under the impact of irradiation, and that is believed to be one of the reasons irradiation cancer treatment debilitates you and has such bad side effects. Irradiation does not have to be by X ray; there is irradiation all over the earth—natural background radiation and cosmic radiation, which nobody escapes. We get quite a bath of that in a steel building. (Did you know if you raise rats under a lead roof they have less cancer?)

There are fats within the human cell, in the membrane and the cell wall. When irradiation hits the fats in the cell, what goes on is comparable to what happens to a bottle of vegetable oil that is stored in a warm pantry and turns rancid. The fat in the cell and the fat in the cell wall can, in a sense, become rancid. This process releases energetic molecules that have no right to be loose within the human body. They are called free radicals.

58

A free radical acts like a billiard ball thrown on a table where there are a lot of other billiard balls; the first one hits the second and the second hits the third, and you get a chain reaction. In the course of that chain reaction an interior wall of a cell—more correctly a little bag within the cell called the lysosome—may be penetrated by the free radical that has been released by the attack of oxygen on the fats in the cell or in the cell wall. The lysosome is like a garbage disposal—it has highly selective active enzymes inside and when the free radical penetrates the wall of that lysosome, those enzymes spill out into the cell. Now, instead of digesting garbage, they are digesting the cell.

In the last ten years you have probably lost 1 percent of your brain cells by this process. It is a process that goes on in us all the time and it is a step toward accelerated aging. Now, if you will remember that the incidence of cancer is concomitant with aging—there tends to be more cancer as we grow older—you will understand why we regard these free radicals as threatening us not only with premature aging or accelerated aging but with the formation of cancer-producing substances in the body. None of this is based on pure supposition. There is a type of fat that has been found in very old people on autopsy and that is always considered to be "senile fat." That same fat has been produced in young animals, so it is not caused by aging but by withholding the biological antioxidants, like vitamin C and vitamin E, which should be in their diets. Thus we have some evidence, but evidence does not convince the medical establishment.

For many years we have been aware that vitamin E was a potent antioxidant; recently we were made aware that this explains the beneficial effects of vitamin E on the heart. Then we became aware that selenium is an antioxidant and that explains part of its usefulness, at least as an antiaging factor, as a factor to prevent damage to the heart during a heart attack, and as a factor that may prevent similar types of damage from free radical activity in arthritis and other disorders. The list of antioxidants, beginning back in 1960, has been growing: glutathione, citrus bioflavonoids, inositol, choline, carotene, vitamin C.

One of the newer antioxidants to be discovered comes from an astonishing source, as documented in a report from the University of Tokyo entitled "The Antioxidant Effect of Sweet Potato." A methanol extract of a small amount of freeze-dried sweet potato was found to have markedly strong antioxidant activity, equivalent to a substantial amount of vitamin E. When the major phenols extracted from the sweet potato were tested for antioxidant activity, their effect was weaker than that of the extract of sweet potato. The researchers tried combining the phenols with some of the amino acids found in sweet potatoes and found that although the amino acids by themselves had very little antioxidant activity, the combination of the phenols with the amino acids had a great deal of activity. They claim there is some synergistic action of the phenols and the amino acids that is responsible for the sweet potato's antioxidant properties.

Antioxidants are antiaging, they are anticancer, and they stimulate the immune system. There are also inflammatory properties in vitamin E and selenium. When good antioxidant activity is found in a staple food, it is good news. For instance, both brewer's yeast and fish are excellent sources of the antioxidant selenium.

Selenium. Selenium may help protect against heart attacks, is an antiaging factor, and protects against more types of cancer than any other single agent ever identified.

When animals are treated with any of a wide range of carcinogens (cancer-causing chemicals), the addition of selenium to their normal diet significantly reduces the number of resulting tumors. Also, selenium supplementation inhibits certain spontaneous tumors linked with viruses in animals. There is a link between viruses and cancers, and a protective link between selenium and the type of tumor that is caused by viruses. In several human population studies, estimated dietary selenium intake in states and cities of the United States, as well as internationally, has correlated inversely with death rates from common cancers such as those of the breast, colon, lung, and pancreas. Where selenium levels were low, cancers of the breast, colon, lung, and pancreas were more frequent. The opposite was also true: Where selenium levels were higher, cancers of the breast, colon, lung, and pancreas were less frequent.

Women with breast cancer tend to have low levels of selenium; women without cancer tend to have higher levels. The crowning irony is that in areas of the world where women have more breast cancer because their intake of selenium is low, farmers are told to give selenium to chickens and cattle.

In one study of the relationship between selenium intake and incidence of cancer, American subjects with the lowest levels of selenium in the group were found to have twice the risk of cancer as compared with those whose selenium intake was at the highest level in the group. This evidence suggests that increased intake of selenium might reduce the incidence of human cancer.

Sometimes a milligram (a thirtieth of an ounce) or a microgram (a thousandth of a milligram) offers protection. If you don't think nutrients play a role in these microscopic quantities, you have never read the literature on the interrelationshp between selenium intake and susceptibility to certain types of cancer.

Selenium affects the immune system. That's the system you want functioning at its best possible level to protect you against bacteria, viruses, and cancers.

I once read an article in a newspaper in which a nutritionist (I don't know what his qualifications were) was quoted as saying that Carlton Fredericks was recklessly telling the public to increase selenium intake. Selenium, he said, is highly toxic. Here is the old problem of language. There is no such thing as a toxic substance; there is only a toxic dose. On the air, as elsewhere, I recommend a maximum of 200 micrograms of selenium daily as a supplement to the American diet. How did I arrive at that "reckless" figure? The Japanese woman (with a high resistance to breast cancer) averages about 500 micrograms a day on her usual diet of fish. The American woman averages between 200 and 250 micrograms. So, if I say add 200 micrograms as a supplement, this brings you up to the Japanese level. At last report, the Japanese population was flourishing; the 500-microgram selenium intake has not decimated them.

I pointed out before that in areas where there is a deficit of selenium in the soil (and therefore a deficit is likely to be present in the animals), the cattle breeders and the chicken raisers are advised to give their animals supplements of selenium or to bring in feed from other areas where the selenium value in the soil is higher in order to keep the animals healthy. That's why eggs are a good source of selenium.

In those areas where the selenium value is low, women have lower blood values for selenium and more breast cancer. Breast cancer and low selenium go hand in hand. Healthier women have higher levels. Unfortunately, there are no bulletins for the women in these areas that say: "We are giving the cattle and chickens selenium supplements. Are you taking care of yourself?" I want you to take care of yourself!

What are the appropriate sources of selenium in the diet and what are the appropriate forms of selenium supplementation?

Selenium linked with methionine seems to be the predominant form of selenium found in wheat and other natural foods. The content is reduced, however, when the foods are overprocessed, so wheat that you buy in the form of white bread is no longer a good source of selenium. The same is true of white rice, white flour, degerminated cornmeal, processed rye, processed buckwheat, etc. The organic, food-derived forms of selenium have good efficacy in the body; they're well absorbed and they're stable. The removal of this particularly effective form of selenium from processed foods has prompted the development of a type of yeast that is high in selenium as a commercial supplementary source, and it has been shown to be rich in methionine bound with the selenium. It reproduces the usable form of selenium found in food. This form of selenium is thought to be substantially less toxic than selenium from sodium selenite, the other common form of selenium. In the body, these two forms are roughly equivalent in efficacy, but the therapeutic index, or activity, of the food form seems to be considerably superior to the sodium selenite form.

I recommend the yeast-bound selenium as a supplement. In the body the selenium methionine—the food form used in this yeast—can be incorporated directly into the proteins the body manufactures. This constitutes a kind of time-release form from which the body can extract selenium as it needs it over a period of time. The food form of selenium would seem more appropriate than the organic form.

Vitamin C. Many of you think that you know the story of vitamin C. I doubt very much that you know the entire story. Very few people do. But, having the long perspective, I'm acquainted with it. I'm going to give you as much as I can of the real story, including the heartbreaking tale of the blockage of research in the application of vitamin C to cancer.

The abnormal cells characteristic of cancer are constantly being made in the body, but what keeps us from developing the full-blown disease is the wide array of tumor cell destroyers that circulate around the body constantly. It has been shown by Griffiths and colleagues that about 50 percent of patients about to undergo surgery for cancer of the colon or rectum have malignant cells circulating about the body through the bloodstream. Yet many of these patients survive. Since there is no recurrence of the cancer in them, it is obvious that the circulating malignant cells were somehow destroyed. The question is how? Well, you know the answer: The patient's immune system acts as a search-and-destroy agency. These defenders are largely dependent on vitamin C, and in addition to that, vitamin C seems to combat malignancy directly. Two researchers, Benedict and Jones, at the Children's Hospital in Los

63

Angeles examined the effect of ascorbic acid on mouse embryo cells that had been exposed to cancer-causing agents. The transformation of the cells into cancerous ones was completely blocked for as long as twenty-three days. Even after the cells had transformed to a tumorlike state, vitamin C caused 75 percent of them to revert to normal.

Another study, the results of which I have applied clinically, was conducted by Dr. Mary Poydock, professor of biology and director of cancer research at Mercyhurst College in Erie, Pennsylvania, and associates at the St. Thomas Institute in Cincinnati, Ohio. In a series of experiments *in vitro* and in living animals, they found that a combination of vitamin C and vitamin B_{12} (they named the combination Mercytamin) definitely inhibits the division of cancer cells without affecting normal ones. Higher doses of vitamin C alone showed some action in that direction, but the researchers reported that vitamin C and vitamin B_{12} in combination are effective against sarcoma, carcinoma, and leukemia. (Dr. Victor Herbert claimed if you took vitamin C you destroyed your B_{12}; his paper was refuted by several competent researchers. Dr. Poydock's research gives solid evidence that vitamins C and B_{12} actually work together.)

These are animal studies; what about people? A University of Kansas Medical Center group headed by Chan H. Park showed that vitamin C can suppress the growth of leukemic cells in humans. When weak concentrations of vitamin C were added to the culture medium, the number of leukemic cell colonies was reduced by 21 percent with no damage to the normal precursors of those cells in the bone marrow. French scientists and a group at Baylor University School of Medicine demonstrated that vitamin C is toxic to malignant melanoma cells from human beings. The addition of tissue saturation concentrations to the cell culture resulted in a 50-percent decrease in the formation of cancer colonies.

Not all the work has been done only in the test tube. Dr. Robert Yanomoto, director of surgical laboratories at City of Hope National

Medical Center in California, along with two colleagues from the National Cancer Institute, did research with healthy young adults who were given five grams of vitamin C daily for three days. In response, lymphocyte blastogenesis—cell division causing the rapid multiplication of a type of white blood cell that defends against cancer—increased significantly. When the dose of vitamin C was increased to ten grams for three days, the rate of lymphocyte blastogenesis was even greater. Researchers have shown that the genesis of these cells that help us fight off cancer becomes more and more impaired as cancer advances, and the state of this mechanism should correlate well with the prognosis for the patient. In a seemingly healthy person, you give a diet low in vitamin C, watch the cell division of the cancer-combatting white cells, and thereby estimate the susceptibility to cancer for the patient.

Jorgen Schlegel and his associates at Tulane University School of Medicine demonstrated that substances commonly found in human urine may cause cancer in the urinary tract. Researchers believe that the oxygen-scavenging action of vitamin C can block these substances from reacting with oxygen so they are not transformed into carcinogens. Dr. Schlegel now routinely gives one thousand to fifteen hundred milligrams of vitamin C—enough to exceed the body's requirements so vitamin C spills into the urine—daily to patients with bladder tumors who are in a high-risk category due to smoking or drinking large amounts of coffee, cola, or alcohol. When this state is maintained, no new bladder cancers develop.

The effect of vitamin C on cervical cancer was investigated by a team headed by Sylvia Wasserfield Smoller at the Johns Hopkins University School of Hygiene and Public Health. There were 169 women involved in the study: 87 of the women had cervical dysplasia (cell abnormality) detected by Pap smears; 82 of the women had normal Pap smears. Variables such as age and sexual activity were taken into consideration and matched pairs of women—one with cervical dysplasia and one without—were compared. It was found that when the vitamin C intake was below the level of the

USRDA (60 milligrams) there was a tenfold increase in the risk of cervical dysplasia. In the United States, 35 percent of menstruating women have a daily intake of less than thirty milligrams of vitamin C; 68 percent have a daily intake of less than eighty-eight milligrams. These women are at increased risk of developing cervical dysplasia—and therefore, cervical cancer—and would benefit from an increase in their vitamin C intake.

Vitamin E. In a study some years ago samples of blood plasma were taken from five thousand women between the ages of twenty-eight and seventy-five and then frozen. Seven years later, thirty-nine of the women had developed breast cancer. Vitamin levels in their blood plasma were compared with the vitamin levels in plasma from seventy-eight matched controls (women in the same group who did not develop breast cancer and were in the same age distribution). The vitamin A (retinol) levels were no different, but the breast cancer victims had significantly lower levels of vitamin E and somewhat lower levels of beta carotene than the controls. The risk of breast cancer was found to be 5.2 times higher for the women with the lowest vitamin E levels and 2.8 times higher for the women with the lowest beta carotene levels than for those with the highest vitamin E and beta carotene levels.

The important antioxidant vitamin E is available in several forms: alpha, beta, delta, and gamma tocopherol. Alpha tocopherol is the most active form of vitamin E in the cell, but it does not have the most satisfactory antioxidant activity. In fact, alpha tocopherol has the least antioxidant value. Delta tocopheral has the most antioxidant activity, followed by the gamma form and then the beta form. If you want the best antioxidant effect from vitamin E, it is best to get "mixed" tocopherols containing several (if not all) of the forms.

Available antioxidant preparations are often intended for chemically hypersensitive people and so do not include those antioxidants derived from or belonging to families that cause allergenic reactions in sensitive people.

If you do not have those sensitivities you should supplement the combined antioxidants formula with choline and inositol, one thousand milligrams each, three thousand milligrams of the citrus bioflavonoids, and one thousand milligrams of L cysteine in addition to that which is contained in the combined formula. Cysteine is a sulfur-containing amino acid and is probably more likely to disturb allergic people than any other protein acid, so although included in combined antioxidant formulas it is only in a very small amount.

A typical acceptable (though not entirely useful) formula would contain glutathione; L cysteine (rather than cystine), for getting mercury out of the body; ascorbic acid (vitamin C) made from Sago palm, to avoid corn allergy, as most vitamin C comes from corn; vitamin B_1; vitamin B_2; pantothenic acid (vitamin B_5); vitamin B_6 as pyridoxil 5 phosphate; beta carotene (vegetable vitamin A); dl-alpha tocopherol (a form of vitamin E), a nonallergenic synthetic; zinc sulfate; sodium selenite (selenium), not as well utilized as that from yeast but less allergenic; and niacinamide.

You may note lecithin is omitted here, because it comes from soy. The citrus bioflavonoids are omitted because some people are sensitive to citrus. My experience has been that most people who are sensitive to citrus fruit can use the bioflavonoids because they are made from the white matter on the inside of the peel. Along with paraaminobenzoic acid that is the type of formula that is antiaging, anticancer, and a bolster to the immune system. All told, a pretty nice series of actions.

It's not, however, a panacea; it does not do the same job for everybody, and it does not do it to the same extent for everybody. Given the absence of allergic reaction to the nutrients, I would say no one fails to derive some benefit from this type of formulation. A combined antioxidant formulation such as this is a way to avoid taking many different capsules of different nutrients simultaneously and probably saves money too.

Breast Cancer

Japanese women have a high resistance to breast cancer when they are living in Japan, but when they come to the United States they lose that resistance. In changing from the Japanese to the American diet, the Japanese woman drops her selenium intake by 40 to 50 percent! Seafood, a staple of the Japanese diet but not of the American diet, is rich in selenium. Selenium intake is, as we have seen, inversely related to the incidence of certain types of cancer, particularly breast cancer.

There is a physician in Cleveland who says the answer to the problem of breast cancer is to castrate all women at age thirty-eight. (Prostate cancer being to men what breast cancer is to women, I suggested to him castrating all men at age thirty-eight in the name of prophylaxis. I didn't get an enthusiastic response on that.) A researcher at the University of Texas had another remedy: Remove the breast tissue of newborn female babies at birth. (He said he realized this would cause some problems. It is a simple operation, but growing up breastless might prove disturbing. And I want to know what will she do when she wants to nurse her babies and give them the benefit of the immunity of breast milk?)

Breast cancer attacks at an epidemic rate; according to the National Women's Health Network the death rate from breast cancer has remained the same since 1930 despite today's expensive and often traumatic radical surgery, which has not been shown to do any better than less radical surgery plus radiation. Nor have drugs and radiation lowered the death rate. Over a quarter of a million women in this country have breast cancer; more than a hundred thousand are diagnosed in a year; as many as thirty-three thousand of those will die. We have an epidemic of this disease, and it is a bad one.

There are several ways to find out if a breast lump is malignant or benign. Probably the only way your physician would trust is a biopsy. The physician will judge by position, by whether the lump is fixed or movable, by the appearance of the other breast tissue, and if he's not happy with his findings he'll confirm with a biopsy. One of the reasons for this procedure is that the public sues for malpractice so readily these days that the doctor must practice defensive medicine and cover all bases.

The radical mastectomy—the mastectomy in which a cut was made all the way over to the underarm area—was performed for nearly ninety years without adequate testing. When they finally tested they discovered they didn't have to do radical mastectomies on a large percentage of the women who ordinarily are subjected to the mutilation, pain, and disability it causes. They found they could use a lumpectomy followed by irradiation—a much gentler approach, however much you may not like irradiation, and one that's still better than a radical mastectomy.

I have used another procedure. I have had the immune system studied because there is at least one immune factor that is produced only when there is cancer present and you can identify that factor. Well, this is the same story: Good nutrition does not help cancer grow. It helps the patient; it doesn't block chemotherapy.

Dr. Linus Pauling has said, "Of all the possible ways known to me to make progress against cancer in the next decade or two, the use of natural substances will, in my view, turn out to be the most important." In the years before the National Cancer Institute's decision to pour millions of dollars into research and prevention programs using "natural inhibitors," namely vitamins, Dr. Pauling had made eight applications to that Institute to further his research on vitamin C and cancer, and he met with eight refusals. Nutrition offers a great deal of promise and at long last is recognized as helping to prevent breast cancer.

Let me pass on this note which came to me as a result of a broadcast I made on national radio:

> This is a note of thanks for your book *The Nutrition Guide*, which was brought to my attention by you during

an interview on the radio. I had a fibroid breast and the beginning of the same in the other breast. My ob-gyn in San Leandro [California] examined me on December 8 and insisted on mammography. On December 9 the radiologist reported there were no malignancies. Nevertheless, my doctor suggested that I see a breast surgeon for removal of some of the tissue. Needless to say, I was relieved to hear "no malignancies," but my sister's terminal cancer began in the breast, and I initiated your suggested nutritional program on December 10. On December 17 I started my first menstrual period in three and a half months. Today one breast is clear of fibroid tissue; the pressure in the other one is greatly decreased. I know you have explained that this nutritional program may take months but in my case there is remarkable improvement in just sixteen days. I have one problem with the [nutritional] program: I cannot find a headache remedy and am forced to use pills.

Choline and inositol come in equal parts, so I am taking a thousand milligrams of each rather than the suggested five hundred milligrams of inositol and one thousand of choline. It is impossible to find B complex without PABA, so I do have to take ninety milligrams of PABA a day.

Here she is referring to the supplementary doses of choline and inositol, not a therapeutic dose. Let me explain why she is concerned about the PABA in the vitamin B complex preparation. PABA stimulates the body's estrogen activity, and it is that activity which we are trying to quiet down when a woman has cystic breast disease. So, this woman went out to look for a vitamin B complex preparation without PABA. I would be satisfied if the preparation had up to thirty milligrams of PABA. Ninety milligrams is too high, and there are vitamin B complex preparations on the market that have the lower amount.

In the process of controlling estrogen, you are helping yourself to avoid cystic breast disease, uterine fibroid tumors, and endometriosis, all of which are sometimes reversed with therapeutic doses of the right nutrients, but as I've said before, you are also helping to make menstruation more tolerable.

The letter continues:

> This was my first menstrual period in thirty-three years with no cramps. I am truly writing to thank you, but if I can help you in any way, I offer you my time. Female problems are so often ignored by male doctors. I'm not a women's libber, only a woman experienced with male doctors. One male doctor wanted to remove my uterus to control bleeding. I told him, "Let's wait. I'm rather attached to my uterus and I'd like to keep it." I'm very serious in my offer to help. I'm a woman employed in a man's field. Female medical problems are frowned upon. You have helped me in many, many ways.

Now you multiply that letter—and I'm not exaggerating, I'm being conservative—by maybe ten thousand over the past ten to twenty years, and you will understand the emphasis I have placed on control of female hormone metabolism as an aid to women in coping with problems that are considered the inevitable price for the biological birthright of being female and able to reproduce. Those problems are not unavoidable and they obviously can be coped with. The nutritional protocol is not a panacea. There are failures. There have been many successes.

Garlic and Cancer

When I looked into the literature, in the *American Journal of Chinese Medicine* (which gives you some idea how far afield one has to go to pick up information in these areas), I found an animal experiment with amino acids (the building blocks of protein), garlic, and cancer. What they did was measure proliferation of cancer cells after ten days on diets supplemented with garlic or with individual amino acids. Those animals that received garlic had a decrease in the incidence of cancer of 20 percent to 51 percent. The amount of garlic given to the animals was large, 0.6 grams per day to a small mouse. I don't think this is a tenable method of preventing cancer, but it does indicate garlic has some actions we do not ordinarily anticipate. There was also a 50 percent inhibition of cancer produced by varying doses of methionine, lysine, and histadine. That must come as a shock to the people who tell you that you must cut down on protein if you want to avoid cancer. This report shows exactly the opposite.

High Protein, High Fat, or High Sugar?

In the late seventies and early eighties there was a series of studies that tended to show, in the opinion of the authors, that high protein is identified with increased breast cancer. When I first read these reports I thought, for a number of cogent reasons, these people must be out of their minds. If high protein is responsible for breast cancer, there shouldn't be an Eskimo woman left alive. There shouldn't be a Masai or Mongolian woman left alive. I can go on; the list of ethnic groups on high-protein diets would be long. It includes Georgians, the Russians who have the reputation for all living to be ninety or a hundred years old. Nathan Pritikin once remarked publicly that no high-protein group has a long life span. He simply hadn't done his homework.

There's a second reason why these research results amazed me, a reason that is even better than epidemiological evidence. When you look at the diet in a high-protein country, you are automatically looking at a high-fat diet. Where do you find a piece of meat without fat? Where do you find cheese without fat? Milk without fat? The list is endless; I defy you to eat a high-protein diet from natural sources—not a protein concentrate—that is not automatically higher in fat than it is in protein. How do you know, therefore, that protein is the culprit rather than fat?

When you buy a steak or lamb chops and you take the meat home, how do we know what you do with the fat? Some of you trim it off. Some of you cook it. Some of you consume it. Any indictment of fat intake in the American diet is predicated on an estimation, not on an actual measurement, but only a guess of how much fat you are consuming. That's point number one. Point number two: You are told that red meat is bad, but why is white meat good? You know, this goes back to the old diets they used to serve for gastric ulcer. You were told to eat chicken but the white meat only. What's the matter with the dark meat and what's the difference between chicken and beef, between beef and pork, between pork and lamb? This was pure superstition. It was superstition then and it remains that now.

Well, how do you work out a correlation now? How do you say to the public, "You women shouldn't eat protein in the quantities in which you are eating it because it causes breast cancer," because one could take exactly the same data, exactly the same correlation and say, "Hey, wait a minute. Yes, these countries are high protein and the countries which are high protein are higher in fat and how do you know that fat is not responsible?"

In order to establish a link between protein and breast cancer you have to use a correlation to imply causation, something like this: American women eat a lot of meat and Japanese women eat a lot of fish and the Japanese have very little breast cancer and therefore it is our intake of meat that is responsible for our being so susceptible to breast cancer that one American woman in every eleven is going to get it. That is using correlation to imply causation. But here is a good example of the fallacy of this type of thinking: On Monday night you drink whiskey and soda and you get drunk.

The following night you drink gin and soda and get drunk. On the third night you drink vodka and soda and get pie-eyed. Obviously, soda is intoxicating. It is the only constant in the entire picture. That type of reasoning has been used to indict high-fat diets as being responsible for breast cancer, and the indictment of fat rests on the same uneasy foundation that the indictment of protein rests on—because the theory ignores the fact that there are numerous ethnic groups whose diets are high in fat or high in protein or high in both for whom breast cancer is not a threat. The fat–breast cancer link is supposed to be bolstered by the experience of the Japanese women who leave Japan, abandon their high-fish diet, and adopt the American diet. Doing so may or may not change the original fat intake of the individual, but it *certainly* increases the intake of sugar, a fact that has evaded the scrutiny of those researchers who seem obsessed with fats.

Now, let's take it one step beyond that. What countries in the world eat 120 pounds of sugar a year per capita? Not the disadvantaged countries. The countries where large amounts of sugar are consumed are places like England, the United States, France, Germany—the affluent countries.

So, here we have millions of people who are eating high-fat, high-sugar, and high-protein diets, but the scientific researchers come along and decide the high protein is what gives them breast cancer. How do they know? What's the evidence? The chemistry behind the most common types of breast cancer is one that involves sugar, not protein. In fact, in order to interrupt that sugar-related chemistry, I always recommend that women raise the protein in their diet.

When I am faced with a woman who is under the influence of too much female hormone activity—as evidenced in premenstrual symptoms, prolonged menstrual periods, heavy hemorrhaging, breast cysts, uterine fibroids—the first thing I do is make sure she cuts down the sugar and raises the protein in her diet. Those two steps reduce the uncontrolled estrogen activity and work to prevent estrogen-dependent cancer. I don't recommend cutting down the protein alone. I've gotten into friendly arguments with those who say a high-protein diet is a mistake for sufferers of hypoglycemia; but women suffering from low blood sugar will not be straightened out by high carbohydrate intake. The woman with low blood sugar and a dietary history of high carbohydrate intake is often the woman with excessive female hormone activity. She is the woman with cystic mastitis, uterine fibroids, disturbed menstruation, and she is very vulnerable to estrogen-dependent breast cancer, which constitutes one-third of all breast cancers. If this chemistry were interrupted by dietary changes uniformly applied among women throughout the United States, we could save as many as thirty-three thousand lives yearly. These women would otherwise develop breast cancer.

The neglected role of sugar intake in breast cancer has now been scrutinized by competent scientists. In an article titled "Sugary Foods May Promote Breast Cancer," which appeared in the July 1983 issue of *Medical Hypothesis,* Stephen Seely of the University of Manchester and Dr. D. F. Horrobin, well known for his work involving the use of evening primrose oil for premenstrual syndrome, highlight a striking correlation between dietary intake of sugar and mortality from breast cancer. In twenty countries the correlation held!

Suspecting that a disease is linked to diet does not identify the item in the diet that has the toxic property, but dietary pathogens— the disease-causing elements in diet—*can* be traced by looking for a match between the geographical distribution of the disease and the consumption of various foodstuffs. A statistical survey was done that showed that the geographical distribution of breast cancer varies with age—not a surprising discovery for a disease that is hormonal and in which dietary factors overlap. The report stated that it is reasonable to assume that hormonal effects predominate in younger women and dietary factors may become increasingly important in older women. And so the geographical distribution of breast cancer in older women is more likely to point to the offender in the diet which is creating the mischief. This is based on studies of women conducted for a period of ten years. This has a solid foundation. This is not merely guessing at how much fat you're eating. This is not indicting protein on the basis of some experiments with mice. This is actual observation of women. The researchers came to the conclusion that for older women the relationship is almost one-to-one: The more sugar the woman eats the more likely she is to have breast cancer. They came to the inescapable conclusion that sugar consumption is more closely related to mortality from breast cancer than is fat consumption, and that the diet plays a more important role in fatal breast cancer in older women than in younger ones. And since diabetic women are at increased risk for breast cancer, they believe that elevation of insulin production caused by sugar may be the connecting link between sugar intake and breast cancer.

Insulin is a hormone secreted when glucose levels are rising in the blood. The public image of insulin is that it's a digestive enzyme, it's kindly, it's necessary for the metabolism of sugars and starches, which is not, in fact, the case. The public image really distorts what is actually going on. Insulin functioning can be visualized as priority rationing, which in lean seasons determines what tissues can draw sugar. The essential and irreplaceable tissues get first call. When food is plentiful, there is enough insulin to satisfy the needs of all the organs. At times when food is scarce, some of the organs will be starved. (The female breast is very low in the order of priorities.) Insulin is a requirement for the growth of breast tissue, and breast cancer cells, at least initially, are dependent on it. Its connection with breast cancer is essentially the same as that of estrogen and prolactin, another hormone. Commercial refined sugar consists of glucose and fructose. They're split in the digestive tract and when they're split apart the glucose immediately enters the circulation. The fructose is inverted, converted into glucose in the liver, and it follows, but after a brief interval. The sudden appearance of glucose in the bloodstream, the sudden rise of the blood glucose level, evokes a quick response. The pancreas produces insulin and this results in an overabundance of insulin and one of the results, of course, could be low blood sugar. According to this argument, glucose is a supersugar and when consumed as such its entry into the bloodstream is not preceded by any work on the part of the metabolism. Glucose is used by the food industry mainly in the manufacture of confections. In Britain and the Netherlands it accounts for about 10 percent of the total consumption of sugar, in Ireland 8 percent, in Germany and France 5 percent. The largest consumers of glucose are the nations that have the highest rate of death from breast cancer.

There is chemical logic to what I'm saying; there is no chemical logic to the linkage between protein and breast cancer. Estrogen and substances in plant foods that mimic estrogen can interact with naturally produced hormones and so promote breast cancer. What substances mimic the action of estrogen in natural foods? One is in legumes—peas and beans. The most common legumes in pasture plants are clover and soybeans. Sheep are particularly sensitive to these estrogen-mimicking compounds, presumably because they crop the pastures more closely than cows. If the sheep get an overdose of the plant estrogens, they experience infertility, difficult labor, and difficult lactation. Estrogen can have an indirect effect on the breast even when it is an estrogen-mimicking substance from plants. Yet countries where a lot of sugar is eaten have high breast cancer; countries where a lot of peas and beans are eaten have less breast cancer, even though the logic does not dictate that those are the findings. But you need to note the age of the women, because that is another variable: In the countries where the consumption of peas and beans is negatively linked with breast cancer in young women, it is more prevalent than in older women. In Japan, for instance, breast cancer mortality in the sixty-five and up age group is 14 percent. In Britain, in the thirty-five to forty-four age group, it is 36 percent.

Now we come back to the chemistry I've already mentioned. The higher the consumption of sugar, the more insulin is released in the body as a consequence, and the more you are likely to disturb the delicate mechanism that keeps estrogen under control. Remember the hormone we're dealing with: If we give estrogen to a seventy-year-old woman, she will stain as though a menstrual period were starting. You're talking about biological dynamite.

The findings of these researchers confirm absolutely what I have observed in decade after decade of the application of diet in reducing stimulation of the breasts by estrogen. I have been able to halt or reverse estrogen-dependent cystic breast disease with a high-protein, high-fat diet that is low in sugar. No matter where we set the fat intake, the treatment is unsuccessful if the patients continue to maintain the American level of sugar intake. This averages a teaspoonful every thirty to thirty-five minutes, twenty-four hours a day—unbelievable! Vitamin B complex intake is an important factor, too; it adds to the indictment of sugar because sugar increases the need for B vitamins while diminishing the supply.

In another study it was found that the urinary excretion of estrogen was higher in vegetarians. That means vegetarian women get rid of their estrogen—or some of it—by excretion. The omnivorous woman tends to retain more, which means the estrogen that might otherwise be excreted is reabsorbed. Now, I don't know precisely how to interpret this, but I'll give you one interpretation. There is a higher fiber content in the vegetarian diet than in the average mixed diet of the omnivorous woman. A high-fiber diet speeds up the transit time for food to be digested and the residues to be excreted. If you speed that up there is less time for anything to be reabsorbed, and this may well explain the lower incidence of breast and uterine cancer and of endometriosis in vegetarian women. But, the difference is not going to be found in the protein intake of the two groups. The allegation that protein is responsible for breast cancer I regard as one of those theories that go through the newspapers and other media, attract a lot of attention, and disappear from sight. We have millions of years of experience with meat, with fat, with other sources of protein and fat—all the way back to the days of hunting, herding, and gathering. The dietary newcomer is the 120 pounds of sugar a year.

The mechanism that protects you from estrogenic hormone is in the liver, and that mechanism is diet dependent. If you don't eat properly it won't work. You want to wreak havoc on that mechanism? Eat plenty of sugar. Fat and protein don't harm that mechanism. Sugar, caffeine, and overprocessed foods deprived of vitamin B complex do.

Let us take a look at what is going on when wheat is turned into flour. One hundred pounds of grain does not yield one hundred pounds of flour, not even if it is going to be whole wheat flour. There is a certain amount of debris in processed wheat that is too rough for human consumption, and so out of one hundred pounds of wheat you may get eighty-eight to ninety-two pounds of flour. This is one of the reasons for the great differences in texture of whole-grain products. If the wheat has been "stone ground," however, virtually everything that was in the grain goes into the flour, because there is no way to separate the wheat from the chaff in stone grinding.

In ordinary roller mill processing, you can separate out whatever you want to. The wheat germ goes out in one direction, the bran goes out in another. You can get rid of what you want and keep what you want. Out of one hundred pounds of wheat the public gets seventy-two pounds of flour—that is called 72 percent extraction. The other twenty-eight pounds largely goes into feed for animals, with the result that the animals are being fed better than humans. We say to the industry, "This is wrong," and the food industry replies, "This is what the public wants." But we are trying to change what the public wants.

I haven't seen the industry change yet. In fact, there are ads on television for good nutrition that say you don't have to eat whole wheat if you are eating a balanced diet. Translation: If your diet supplies what we have taken out of our bread, then you can eat our bread.

I'll buy whole wheat. We said to the industry, "Why don't you stop making 72 percent extraction flour? Why not bring it up to 80 percent?" There is good reason for this suggestion: When they come up 8 percent (when they get eighty pounds of flour rather than seventy-two out of a hundred pounds of wheat), the nutritional gain is out of proportion to the 8 percent. You don't pick up just 8 percent more nutrients. You pick up a lot more and it differs for each nutrient. The industry says the public wouldn't accept it. Yet, during the latter part of World War II, when it became obvious we would have to feed starving people released from concentration camps and populations who had been under blockade, this country went to 80 percent extraction at the request of our government so there would be more flour per hundred pounds of wheat, enabling us to feed more people. The industry did it, and we ate it, and I'll bet if you were around then you didn't even know the difference! The bread had a little more color, it was creamier, and that was about all you would notice.

I eat a slice of whole wheat bread with each meal. Is that enough? No. The eternal battle between the waistline and the nutrient requirements is what you are facing. That is why I use special-purpose foods; that is why I use supplements, because I can bring in more nutrients with fewer calories while the food industry is concentrating on calories at the expense of nutrients. They are doing the opposite of what we need and only your vote at the checkout counter will make them change.

Nutrients as Preventive Agents in Cancer

Herbert Spencer once said, "There is a principle which is proof against all information, which is proof against all arguments, which cannot fail to keep a man in everlasting ignorance, and that principle is contempt prior to investigation." That is the picture I saw as I watched the government agencies and the cancer institutions busy testing vitamin A and carotene and vitamin C and selenium in the treatment or prevention of cancer while very deftly forgetting that it was only a couple of years since they were calling us nutritionists quacks for making the suggestion that these nutrients might have that kind of usefulness. In Australia vitamin A was studied in twenty patients who had cancer of the head and neck; twenty healthy volunteers served as controls. In the tumor patients, serum levels of vitamin A were significantly lower than in the controls and the dark adaptation (the eyesight of the individual in its adjustment to a change in illumination from bright to dark) was disturbed, an effect that occurs only after vitamin A deficiency is of long duration.

I could give you a hundred of those examples because the literature is full of them today—carotene (the vegetable form of vitamin A) is now endorsed as a possible preventive for cancer; selenium and vitamin C similarly. Has orthodox medical treatment for cancer been so effective?

Ivan Illich wrote: "I do not know that, in the overwhelming majority of cancers where a lot of money has been spent on diagnosis and therapy, either the precocity of the diagnosis or the kind of treatment has had any impact on the survival rates. . . . We do have increasing evidence that those who are treated supposedly for curative purposes, at best, have an earlier onset of anguish, a prolonged period of impairment, and a greater intensity of pain than those who succeed in escaping the doctor." And Doctor Hardin Jones of the University of California Department of Medical Physics, describing the dividends from orthodox cancer treatment, said: "My studies have proved conclusively that untreated cancer patients actually live up to four times longer than treated individuals. For a typical type of cancer, people who refuse treatment live for an average of twelve and a half years. Those who accepted surgery and other kinds of treatment lived an average of only three years. I

81

attribute this to the traumatic effect of surgery on the body's natural defense mechanisms—the body has a natural defense against every type of cancer. Medical treatment seems to interfere with and mess up this natural resistance. You see, it is not the cancer that kills the victim. It is the breakdown of the defense mechanism that eventually brings death. With every cancer patient who keeps in excellent physical shape and boosts his health to build up his natural resistance, there is a high chance that the body will find its own defense against cancer."

Do you remember President Richard Nixon declaring war on cancer? By 1978, with two billion dollars spent through the National Cancer Act of 1971, no significant results had yet been brought forth. Still, when cured cancer victims reported they were helped by nutritional therapy, physicians and cancer researchers laughed. Richard A. Passwater, Ph.D., in his book *Cancer and Its Nutritional Therapies,* wrote: "We have paid for all this fruitless research and cover-up. Isn't it time to increase research efforts into nutritional therapies? Public pressure must be brought to bear on those controlling the funding for such programs. Will we continue to allow more than 90 percent of the tax dollars to be used for cancer research that tries to find cancer viruses and develops poisonous drugs as 'therapy' when we already know that at least 90 percent of the cancers are caused by environmental and food pollutants?"

Maybe you think that he exaggerated. He didn't, and I am going to tell you a story of one executive. I heard what I am about to tell you directly from him. One of his children developed a type of cancer, Hodgkin's disease. The child was taken to Sloan-Kettering, where she endured chemotherapy and irradiation. A few weeks later she was described as being in total remission. Her father took her home. The following weekend he and his wife went away for a weekend vacation after the long ordeal and they left their daughter playing tennis. She had a slight case of the sniffles, nothing else on the horizon. Their vacation weekend was interrupted by an emergency telephone call to come home. They returned home to find their daughter dying of pneumonia. She did die. They went back to Sloan-Kettering and talked to the oncologists who had administered the treatment and they asked how did this happen? How did a cold in the morning develop into fatal pneumonia?

The doctor was honest and explicit. He told them it was because the treatment knocks the hell out of the body's defenses, the immune system. With no defense, a small cold becomes a fulminating and lethal pneumonia. That is a side of the picture you don't very often hear about. Nor do you hear about the cancers secondary to the treatment—meaning that irradiation used to treat the cancer may also cause cancer. What you *have* heard over the years is a lot of ridicule of these "crackpots" who recommend nutritional therapy or nutritional prophylaxis for cancer.

I'm not saying you should substitute nutritional therapy for the usual traditional type of cancer treatment. I'm saying you should use nutrition to offset the side effects of chemotherapy and irradiation. For that purpose nutrients have been prescribed, but there is an unexpected dividend for the patient—patients respond to chemotherapy and to irradiation therapy with much more impact on the cancer than would be anticipated. I had the experience of watching that thesis put into action and I have seen it confirmed.

The work on nutrition in the prevention and treatment of cancer has piled up. I pursued a calculated course in supplying information to oncologists on the use of nutrients to offset the side effects of chemotherapy and irradiation. This is not an original idea on my part. I simply implemented it, as I believe nobody else did, because it is recognized that both radiation and chemotherapy create free radicals in the body. These are highly energetic, abnormal compounds (actually abnormal molecules or fragments of molecules) that do a great deal of damage resulting in side effects. If you supply the patient with free radical "quenchers," you may be able to take the patient through chemotherapy and irradiation with greatly reduced side effects or none at all. I felt there was a possibility not

83

only of offsetting these side effects but also of making the therapy more effective. That is the way it has worked out, as the following examples indicate.

- There was a case of an acute breakout of leukemia that was being treated with mild doses of chemotherapy, mild because the patient had already been through the drastic doses and had not responded well but responded beautifully when anti- oxidants, free radical "quenchers," were added to the mild doses of the cytotoxic drugs.
- There was a case of ovarian cancer with widespread metas- tasis in which the side effects of intensive chemotherapy and irradiation were minimal and the patient responded to the treatment better than her condition would have led one to expect as a result of the addition of the antioxidants.
- Then there was a case of oat cell carcinoma of the lung, a very resistant type of cancer and the one responsible for many deaths among smokers who develop lung cancer. For this reason, the doctor did not anticipate that radiation was going to be markedly helpful to the patient. With the ad- dition of antioxidants, the irradiation was indeed markedly successful, so much so that the daughter of the patient called me to tell me in pure ecstasy that the doctor had said that seven-eighths of the cancer had disappeared with the irra- diation and he wanted now to focus it sharply (it had been broad beamed) on the remaining amount of cancer to see whether he could get rid of that.

I found myself faced with a very practical difficulty in attempting to cooperate with physicians seeking information concerning the use of antioxidants to offset the side effects of chemotherapy and irradiation. (This shows, by the way, that your physicians have been just as upset as you by the side effects of what they have been compelled to prescribe for cancer.) The difficulty was with "patient compliance." You are not likely to get the cooperation of the patient if you ask her to take fifteen or twenty capsules, pills, or tablets daily. It is understandable when a mild disorder is the target for the treatment but perhaps a little less understandable when you are dealing with something life-threatening such as cancer. How do you get past the patient compliance barrier when you are compelled to give the doctor a list like the following:

vitamin A	paraaminobenzoic acid
carotene	vitamin C
vitamin B_1	vitamin E
vitamin B_2	selenium
niacinamide	glutathione
inositol	lecithin
choline	cysteine

Many of these factors are not available combined, and the only compromise when faced with a patient compliance problem is to use a vitamin B complex supplement, if you can find one reasonably complete in the vitamin B factors in this list. All vitamin B complex preparations contain B_1, B_2, and niacinamide and usually in sufficient potency, but many do not contain inositol and choline, and if they do it is in quantities so small they are useless. As I mentioned earlier, there are now a few formulations of antioxidants available.

When you speak to a woman about the need for some of these factors and the problem is prevention rather than treatment, it is difficult to persuade her to take a dozen separate nutrients on the basis of the fact that she may be a target for breast cancer thirty years from now. The fact that these nutrients are also helpful in premenstrual syndrome, shortening menstrual periods, reversing cystic breast disease and sometimes even uterine fibroids helps to convince her it's worth availing herself of these nutrients.

Antioxidants, in addition to their use in offsetting the side effects of chemotherapy and radiation and in helping women avoid the

85

problems often regarded as the inevitable price of being women, also help to retard the aging process. They are, without exception, antiaging factors.

In the course of putting together my protocol to offset the side effects of conventional cancer treatments, I was puzzled by one thing: We have known since the hydrogen bomb was developed and tested that nutrients can offset the side effects of radiation; animals were deliberately exposed to the radiation. We have learned more about these same nutrients in the last twenty-five years. I'm talking about something very concrete; applying this information may reap some dividends. I would rather you have in your diet the nutrients that are antidotes for oxidizing radiation long before you are subjected to that type of treatment, and I hope you never are.

5 | YEAST INFECTION

Candida is a yeast carried by practically 100 percent of the population. It rests quietly in the body until something tips the system off balance, causing recurring vaginal yeast infections, symptoms of low blood sugar, and multiple allergies.

There is yeast and fungus all around you. When you polish an apple, you are removing fungus. When you eat peanuts, you are eating fungus—there is one variety of African peanut that is actually highly toxic. There is no way to escape fungus and mold. Ordinarily it is balanced in the body by other organisms, unless it is released as the result of a stressful situation and the event is compounded by use of substances that upset the natural chemistry of the body.

Yeast infection very frequently makes itself known as a vaginal infection; there may be soreness or pain during or after sexual relations, burning on urination, itching, or discharge. A physician may prescribe a cream to be applied locally for a week or an antifungus drug in suppository form to kill the fungus. Relief is often temporary and the infection appears again because the yeast is found throughout the body and cannot be cured with local treatment. Candidiasis, an infection caused by the organism *Candida albicans*, is present in vaginal secretions and can be found in up to 15 percent of adult women.

It is possible to get a yeast infection localized in the vagina more or less as a venereal disease, and sometimes without any genital contact. If it's diagnosed promptly, when the local itching, inflammation, and discharge are present, it's possible to get rid of it. Instead of going to powerful antifungus medications that take long to act and may have side effects, many nutritionists first prescribe a local application of yogurt for a localized vaginal infection. The lactobacillus (acid-producing bacteria that ferment yogurt) content of the yogurt can be increased by adding freeze-dried bacteria before application. That is just the beginning of the therapy. The next thing to do is look at how much carbohydrate is being eaten. Overloading on processed carbohydrates will defeat the bacteria in the yogurt. This treatment isn't a panacea, but it is a refreshing change from endless doses of antifungus drugs.

Many women who have recurring monilia infection get a two-week course of treatment. It goes away and a couple of weeks later it's back—or maybe a couple of months go by and the woman gets penicillin or tetracycline for some other infection and then, boom, the monilia is back. Or she takes birth-control pills and develops the infection. It's particularly common, by the way, in diabetics and diabetic families. But, for whatever reason, when this becomes chronic instead of a one-time thing, the reason is that it has entered the intestinal tract and has colonized—usually in the large intestine—and since the opening of the large intestine, the anus, is only an inch or so from the opening of the vagina, cross-infection occurs.

Any time there is irritation in the vagina that reduces the integrity of the mucous membrane lining, the vaginal infection can flare up again. But even when the infection is under control—no symptoms, no signs—if a patient is carrying this yeast in the intestinal tract, and she is allergic to it, then twenty-four hours a day, seven days a week, fifty-two weeks a year, she is in intimate contact with something that is causing her allergic symptoms. That's a terrible stress. It reduces the body's overall resistance. Patients tend to get infections more easily, but most importantly, they begin to get allergic to other things as well. And that's one way candida can pave the way for other allergies.

Let's say a woman has had multiple allergies that have not been responsive to any treatments. She's had a number of vaginal yeast infections, the frequency and severity of which you have not been able to find a logical explanation for. You know she's a victim of candida.

The type of allergy we are talking about is not what most doctors consider allergy. Orthodox medicine recognizes only a limited number of shock organs, those that react allergically. If your nose reacts, you get hay fever; if your eyes react, you get conjunctivitis; if the skin reacts, you get eczema or hives; if the lungs react, you get asthma; and perhaps the intestine could give you some vomiting or pain or diarrhea. That's about it.

It turns out, however, that many patients with allergies have vague and disturbing complaints about their behavior—or other people complain about their behavior. They're irritable, they're nasty, or else they are tired all the time, they have nonspecific problems such as headaches and leg cramps, or frequent urination with no infections. The patient who comes in and whose allergy hasn't even been diagnosed as allergy is often told she's neurotic or that she needs to get away for a vacation, or that she has too many problems.

When a baby is still in the uterus as a fetus, its immune system is programmed so that every protein it comes in contact with is recognized as belonging to it. Therefore its immune system does not react to them abnormally. If the mother is carrying candida and particles of the organism or some of the metabolic by-products get through the placenta into the fetus's circulation, then after birth and for the rest of the child's life it is almost impossible to mount an effective response to this infection.

Recurring vaginal yeast infection is a symptom, it is not the disease. The problem is not local in any one organ, it is body-wide. It involves allergy to the yeast and this in turn may mean other allergies, including allergy to any type of yeast or fungus. The vagina is the target for treatment here, but the problem exists throughout the body. (This is very much like treating tinnitus with therapy directed at the ear when the problem is really in the whole body.)

A candida infection that manifests itself vaginally triggers multiple allergies and allergies trigger low blood sugar. Low blood sugar can initiate allergies or make them worse—you're caught in a vicious circle. You can approach this one-sidedly: for example, treat the low blood sugar to get rid of asthma (in a trial several years ago 25 percent of asthmatics had low blood sugar). But when you approach the problem unilaterally this way you have not solved the problem: If there is candida in the system, the patient is not going to experience total relief. This is an awfully persistent fungus; the immune system does not properly reject it. Treatment should stimulate the immune system to reject the fungus, but the immune system does not recognize it.

There are a great many women who are mistakenly diagnosed as neurotic or psychotic—more frequently neurotic—because they're tired, listless, their spirits are low, they've lost interest in things, are susceptible to infection, have multiple allergies. They wind up in analysis, treated by psychiatrists, and sometimes are dismissed by the internist and the general practitioner with a tranquilizer or antidepressant. Infection, treatment with antifungus or antiyeast drugs, and repeated infection and treatment . . . the history of these women is one of repeated prescriptions for antifungus drugs followed by reinfection.

There are two factors I find consistently associated with recurrent reinfection: multiple allergies and a high-carbohydrate diet. There is a tendency for vaginal yeast infection often to be associated with a high-carbohydrate diet. Behind the localized vaginal yeast infection is body-wide infection with *Candida albicans.*

It makes no sense to treat recurrent vaginal yeast infection as a localized problem. Many medical treatments put stress on the body and render it more susceptible to candida infection—repeated doses of antibiotics, which destroy the useful, friendly bacteria of the intestinal tract; cortisone, which breaks down the body's resistance; birth-control pills. Treatment of candida has not always been successful; it is protracted. But if you don't get rid of the candida, the immune system will be further compromised and multiple allergies will develop.

Once the yeast is triggered, it begins to colonize other tissues. The colon and vagina are favorite targets. When the colon is attacked, the digestive disorders it causes—cramps, gas, and diarrhea alternating with constipation—may be misdiagnosed as irritable bowel syndrome.

Yeast infection can be triggered by antibiotics. Many antibiotics are manufactured by yeast culturing; they come from a fermentation process. They may therefore add to the yeast infection. Antibiotics kill off friendly bacteria, unleashing the organisms they had held in check, killing the bacteria that kept the yeast under control.

Candida albicans is a yeast fungus present in all of us and normally controlled by bacteria in the intestinal tract. When something destroys these bacteria the yeast begins to invade and colonize the body tissues. These yeast colonies release toxins into the bloodstream, causing a variety of symptoms such as lethargy, chronic diarrhea, bladder infections, vaginal yeast infections, cramps, asthma, migraine headache, and severe depression. Usually, candida is thought of as a minor infection of the mucous membranes, skin, and nails. In part, increased use in our culture of antibiotics, steroid hormones, and the birth-control pill allows the candidiasis to become a chronic, systemic infection that causes tissue damage throughout the body. Toxins produced by the candida attack the immune system and as it weakens, the yeast spreads. Many victims appear to have no resistance at all to the yeast infection; the immune system simply does not fight off the disease.

91

To correct candidiasis the antifungus drug nystatin is normally used. The yeast is very stubborn, and treatment may last for several months. The patient should avoid vitamins of yeast origin (many "natural" vitamins are yeast based, particularly the B complex vitamins) and tea, as fungus often grows on the back of tea leaves. There is a type of tea made from the bark of the Brazilian larpacho tree, which does not grow fungus. This tea also appears to destroy candida in much the same way as nystatin.

The patient should follow a low-carbohydrate diet such as is used for treating low blood sugar, no more than sixty to eighty grams of carbohydrate a day. The yeast feeds on carbohydrates—yeast products, sugars, and molds. Antibiotics, steroids, and birth-control pills, which upset hormonal balance, should be avoided.

Lactobacillus, found in yogurt, will destroy candida in the colon. If you are allergic to yogurt you can try eating it only once every four days, which usually allows the body to establish a tolerance. Kyolic, a form of garlic which can be safely eaten in large quantities, will destroy the fungus at the intercellular level where nystatin, because it is not absorbed, cannot reach. Ordinary whole garlic or garlic tablets should not be eaten in large quantities as it shortens the life span of red blood cells.

Vitamin A in large doses—300,000 international units or more to start, later reduced to about 25,000 units of the beta carotene form—is a recommended part of the treatment of candidiasis. Essential fatty acids containing evening primrose oil will help restore the immune system and also fight the candida. Biotin is both a food for the candida organism and an important agent in overcoming it. Large amounts of biotin taken with garlic or the antibiotic nystatin will provide benefits without feeding the fungus.

The orthodox medical protocol for treatment of candidiasis recommends a number of elements that seem to me less beneficial in providing relief and reestablishing the sufferer's health. Supplementation with thymus tissue is meant to help restore the immune system, but the tissue is broken down as it goes through the digestive

92

system. Proteolytic enzymes are recommended, but these too are broken down in the digestive system and large amounts are needed so plenty will be left after digestion to enter the blood and dissolve the candida.

It takes six months to destroy this very stubborn organism. In a person suffering many of the symptoms of low blood sugar—constant tiredness with no apparent cause, multiple allergies, lethargy, insomnia, dizziness, poor concentration, short attention span—but in whom low blood sugar is not present, candidiasis is probably the cause.

The candida yeast loves sugar, and the patient who loves sugar is someone who may develop hypoglycemia, which is known to accompany or trigger many allergies. It is therefore easy to mistake the problem as hypoglycemia when it is actually candidiasis. High intake of sugar may have triggered low blood sugar and encouraged the yeast to invade the body. There is a very useful book on the subject, *The Missing Diagnosis,* by Dr. C. Orian Truss.

Physicians need to catch up with the fields of bioecological allergy and nutrition and patients need to be warned that if they are allergic to yeast and suffer from a yeast infection, they need to avoid vinegar, brewer's yeast, and natural vitamins (they contain yeast); synthetic vitamins are as good as the natural ones. Even psoriasis can result from yeast infection and treatment for the yeast can correct the psoriasis.

Mercury Poisoning from Amalgam Fillings

We have good reason to believe that mercury encourages the candida. We've got to get rid of the mercury to get rid of the yeast. If yeast infection is recognized in a patient, she is put on a strict protocol to get rid of it. But if mercury is present in the body the protocol will not be effective in getting rid of the yeast until the amalgam is removed from the teeth.

Psychosis and insanity have resulted from mercury accumulation in the body as a result of dental fillings. The amalgam used to fill teeth is a mixture of several materials including a large percentage—40 or 50 percent—of mercury. The mercury, in contact with other metals, and in the environment of saliva, which contains salt and other minerals, acts like a battery and generates a current. This results in the release of mercury vapor. The mercury vaporizes over a period of time, accumulating and eventually producing neurological poisoning.

Many of the symptoms of mercury poisoning, such as depression, are overlooked because they seem to be purely emotional. One very frequent physical symptom is low body temperature. This normally indicates an underactive thyroid, but if thyroid medication doesn't help and the temperature stays low, there is a good possibility of mercury poisoning.

Not everyone reacts to mercury. Some people are sensitive and develop symptoms, others do not. But even if you do not show symptoms you could be courting danger. Mercury poisoning is linked to heart attacks. The reason some people react to mercury and others do not is that the sensitivity is similar to allergy. Hypersensitivity to mercury can be tested, but the test carries some hazards. A patch impregnated with mercury is applied to the skin and the patient is placed under observation. If the person is very sensitive to mercury the patch may evoke a terrible reaction.

It is necessary to test whether there is a toxic level of mercury in the body. If that is found, the amalgam must be removed from the teeth. The yeast will retire and multiple allergies may go with it.

The dissimilar metals of amalgam in a wet environment release an electrogalvanic current at the base of the brain. This current, which can be measured, will eventually erode the amalgam and mercury vapor will be released in ever increasing amounts. The vapor will be absorbed by the lungs and travel to the blood, brain, heart, kidneys (where it can be intensely destructive), liver, muscles—the protein in the body. Some dentists can test for electrical activity, which is also believed to be responsible for the pain of temporomandibular joint (TMJ) syndrome. When testing for a current the dentist will determine how much and what kind it is. If removal of the amalgam seems called for, the dentist will also decide in what sequence the amalgam should be removed. The fillings can be replaced with gold or with the composite normally used to fill front teeth, which is less durable than amalgam, or with one of the new types of resins now available and which are safe and durable with a good seal and resistance to abrasion and corrosion.

If the electrical current test shows activity that can lead to corrosion and release of mercury vapor, a mercury vapor test can be done to determine the amount of vapor that may be released. The instrument used to test for the amount of vapor released when you chew can measure with an accuracy down to one microgram.

When a mercury vapor test shows a level being released that is high enough to be of concern, the next step is to test for mercury being carried in the body; a situation that can lead to or contribute to yeast infection. Hair analysis is one approach for determining the presence of mercury in the body. It is not clear, however, if a high level in the hair represents a high level held in the body or a high level being excreted from the body. Generally a baseline is determined from measurements of mercury found not only in the hair but also in the blood and urine. If a high level is found, antimercury nutrients will be given and a month later the blood and urine tests are repeated. The nutrients used contain sulfur because sulfur is an antagonist of mercury. I have seen increases of a factor of forty to sixty of the amount of mercury found in the second test, as the mercury is now being excreted from the body. If the levels are high the treatment is continued.

Glutathione (a protein), selenium, and cysteine (a sulfur-containing amino acid) are all mercury antagonists. A patient is given doses of these for one month and the mercury tests are rerun. In a typical case, the initial tests may show .04 micrograms of mercury in the urine, which is very close to zero. After a month of treatment with the antimercury nutrients a repeat of the test may show a value in the urine of 70 micrograms. Mercury had been being stored in the body tissues and now it is being excreted. We have established the fact that too much mercury is being carried, and treatment is continued.

As treatment is continued the patient will begin to feel worse. This is because as the mercury moves out of the tissues and into the blood the patient begins to feel the effects of the poison. This is temporary, and as the mercury leaves the body the patient will improve.

When the amalgam is removed, exaggerated symptoms of mercury sensitivity may appear temporarily. Headaches become worse, rashes are redder, tempers become hyperirritable. These effects can be moderated with intravenous vitamin C, which increases the permeability of cell walls, allowing the mercury to get out more easily, and attaches to the mercury, helping to take it out of the body. Twenty-one days after the amalgam is removed, the patient is apt to have a bad day. It is necessary to continue supplements of the glutathione, selenium, and cysteine until the accumulated mercury has completely left the body.

The mercury released from amalgam is an efficient mischief maker. It dispossesses zinc from twenty enzymes in the brain. The result can be residual disturbances in zinc, copper, and manganese and in fatty-acid metabolism. Doses of linseed oil or evening primrose oil may be needed to counteract these effects.

Multiple Allergies

A person with multiple allergies—fifty plus allergies, including forty or more to food, some to chemicals, sprays, detergents, household items, perfumes, cologne—would ordinarily be referred to a special isolation facility for treatment. (There is one in Illinois, one in Texas, one in California, one in Florida.) There the patient is put into a stainless-steel room, the air and water are filtered, the people are detoxified, everything the person reacts to is taken away and gradually things are reintroduced, one at a time, so the reaction can be measured. This is a costly procedure and often insurance does not cover it.

If you have had recurring vaginal yeast infections or take birth-control pills or repeated courses of antibiotics or react to mercury from the amalgam in your fillings, a test for candidiasis would be wise. If it is found, treatment of the yeast infection may save you from the need for treatment at an isolation facility. The allergies may be caused by the candidiasis or aggravated by it. In either case, the allergies will be greatly alleviated, if not totally disappear, when the yeast is back under control. Some simple dietary tricks can help also. If milk is brought nearly to a boil and then cooled, often the protein is changed enough for the allergic individual to tolerate it. The same is true of other proteins, which are frequently the key substances in triggering allergy.

Physical symptoms of allergy include the following:

- GENERAL: headache, faintness, dizziness, fullness in the head, excessive drowsiness after eating, insomnia.
- EYE, EAR, NOSE, THROAT: runny or stuffy nose, excessive mucus formation, postnasal drip, watery eyes, blurred vision, earache, ringing or fullness in the ears, fluid in the middle ear, hearing loss, recurrent ear infection, itching ear, ear drainage, sore throat, hoarseness, chronic cough, gagging without apparent cause, canker sores, itching of the roof of the mouth, recurrent sinus trouble.
- HEART, LUNGS: palpitations, arrhythmia, increased heart rate, tachycardia, asthma, chest congestion.
- GASTROINTESTINAL: nausea, vomiting, diarrhea, constipation, bloating, belching, colitis, flatulence, fullness of the stomach, abdominal pain, cramps.

- SKIN: hives, rashes, eczema, dermatitis, pallor.
- OTHER: chronic fatigue, weakness, muscle or joint aches and pain, arthritis, swelling of hands, feet, ankles, extreme urinary frequency or urgency, vaginal itching, vaginal discharge, hunger and binge eating.

The psychological symptoms of allergy include anxiety, panic attacks, depression, crying jags, aggressive behavior abnormal to the personality, irritability, mental dullness, lethargy, confusion, excessive daydreaming, hyperactivity, restlessness, learning disabilities, poor work habits, slurred speech, stuttering, inability to concentrate, indifference, and loss of touch with reality.

Generally speaking, orthodox allergists recognize food, pollen, mold, and some inhalants such as cooking gas as producing allergies. In addition, this list of symptoms can be triggered by antibiotics, in people with hypoglycemia or in women who take birth-control pills, as part of the process leading to candidiasis. You develop multiple allergies you may not be aware of, causing psychological symptoms and symptoms of the head, eyes, ears, nose, throat, heart, lungs, gastrointestinal tract, or skin.

Identifying and Treating Candidiasis

In women the investigation of the causes of multiple allergies goes beyond identifying offending foods, chemicals, drugs, and inhalants. The question of what touched off the multiple allergies must be addressed.

There is much misinformation accepted by unwary medical people, sometimes by unwary nutritionists. Many medical people, believing candida has a "pesky tendency" to reappear in some women— often as a result of prolonged exposure to antibiotics or birth-control pills—follow the standard treatment for the local infection with nystatin or other antifungus drugs and suppositories. They fail to recognize the body-wide nature of the yeast infection.

Treatment of candidiasis by the holistic medical person or medical nutritionist begins with doses of garlic, which has antiyeast properties. Large amounts of biotin, a B complex vitamin, and lactobacillus, the "friendly" bacteria found in milk and yogurt that normally holds yeast in the body in check, are also given. Because yeast loves sugar, a low-carbohydrate diet is part of the treatment. Oral doses of nystatin accompany the treatment. Finally, sensitivity to mercury from amalgam tooth fillings is looked for, as mercury in the body will encourage the yeast in addition to causing many other physical and psychological problems. If an excessive load of mercury is found, the amalgam fillings need to be removed and antimercury nutrients added to the treatment. It may be necessary to bring down the histamine level—not in the blood (this can be taken care of with antihistamine medication) but in the tissues, where it is not brought down by those drugs. Histamine in the tissues can aggravate the systemic tendency to allergy which accompanies candidiasis and can increase symptoms; it can also cause depression. The histamine level in the tissues can be brought down with calcium and methionine. When the candida is body-wide, nutritional treatment can take six months. All these methods are brought to bear on the infection, which orthodox medicine treats only with drugs as a local infection of the genital tract.

It is difficult to tell if a person has systemic candidiasis, but it is easy to test for allergy to yeast. The cytotoxic test is used. The person's blood is exposed to the test substance—tortula yeast, brewer's yeast, and then candida yeast. If the white blood cells swell up or show other abnormal reactions the sample is given an allergy grade of from zero to four—from no allergy to very severe. This test identifies allergy, not infection. A strong reaction to the test for candida allergy would at least be an implication that there is a systemic candida infection.

Mercury poisoning from amalgam tooth fillings is a separate topic, but a frequent combination of circumstances that releases the candida in the body can include depression of the immune system by the mercury. Mercury depresses the immune system, and the immune system is part of the necessary defense against colonization in the body of anything alien, including yeast.

Men get yeast infections but with nothing like the frequency with which they occur in women. There are several reasons why this is so:

- During the menstrual cycle, the increased production of progesterone that follows ovulation results in changes in the vaginal membrane that promote the growth of yeast.
- The birth-control pill, which is also used to treat hormonal imbalances and menstrual irregularities, encourages the growth of yeast.
- Urinary tract problems, which are more common in women than in men, are treated with antibiotics, as are skin problems of teenage girls. These antibiotics also contribute to the growth of yeast.
- The environment of the vagina, warm and dark, provides an ideal home for yeast organisms.
- The hormonal and other changes associated with pregnancy encourage yeast.

A comprehensive picture of the related problems that indicate candida infection will perhaps help you escape being diagnosed as a psychiatric wreck when in fact you are suffering from a physical disorder.

The candida organism can begin to increase in number if your body is under stress or if your immune system has been depressed. When the candida starts to proliferate in the intestinal tract it changes its anatomy and its physiology. It goes from a yeastlike form to a fungus form. The yeastlike state is noninvasive: It's a sugar-fermenting organism. In its fungus state it is invasive, producing long rootlike structures that penetrate the soft tissue of the intestinal tract. The penetration can break down the boundary between the intestinal tract and the rest of the circulation and allows introduction into the bloodstream of substances that may be allergenic. This is why many people with chronic candida overgrowth show a wide variety of allergies. Incompletely digested dietary proteins migrating into the bloodstream can cause a powerful antigenic effect. It's an assault on the immune system.

When as a result of the yeast you absorb incompletely digested protein, you may have endorphinlike activity. Endorphins are the internally produced brain chemicals that control mood, behavior, and memory. The partially digested proteins are called exorphins—produced outside the systemic circulation.

It is a disturbed bacterial flora in the intestinal tract that establishes a favorable environment for the yeast to proliferate. *Lactobacillus acidophilus* cultured from human breast milk can be used to reintroduce friendly bacteria into the bowel, making the intestinal environment less compatible with the growth of the yeast. This had been very successful in reducing candida in the intestinal tract.

Conversion of candida from the yeast to the fungus form is dependent on biotin deficiency, so biotin is administered to discourage the conversion. Oleic acid, which is in olive oil, also interferes with the yeast-to-fungus conversion. Increased fiber, particularly oat bran, is beneficial. Once the candida in fungus form has been converted back to yeast form, healing of the soft tissue of the intestine can be facilitated with high levels of zinc, vitamin A, vitamin E, and calcium pantothenate. Combined with a low-carbohydrate diet, this treatment has been successful in alleviating chronic conditions that were seemingly untreatable in most cases.

6

CONCEPTION, PREGNANCY, AND LACTATION

Reproduction is the ultimate test of nutrition. And yet in this country, in this cornucopia of plenty, infertility is the problem of one couple in every ten. That may come as a shock to you if you've been impressed with all the baby carriages you see, but the fact is that the level of reproductive efficiency in modern American men and women would not be tolerated in stables where they raise thoroughbred horses that have a high cash value.

If we use reproductive efficiency as the test of nutritional well-being, this country is in trouble. Remember, our diets were not planned, they are the product of the happenstance rulings, regulations, and practices of the government, the Department of Agriculture, the dairies, farms, ranches, the processing and packaging industries, the marketplace, and the potent advertising of the food producers. When you consider modern food with its additives, pesticides, residues, and the overprocessing to which it's been subjected, it's not surprising that our nutrition is weakening in supporting reproduction. Yet it is this consideration that is so important in solving the problem of an infertile couple.

I find it paradoxical that when I lectured before the Society for

103

the Investigation of Infertility and Sterility I was the only speaker on the subject of nutrition in some twenty years of programs sponsored by the Society.

If you go to a fertility clinic because you can't conceive, you wind up with the fallopian tubes being inflated and fertility drugs administered, which can lead to multiple births but which fail in many cases. You will not be asked what you eat.

What are the usual recommendations for avoiding infertility? Get rid of your IUD, as it can cause inflammation that might lead to infertility; have an annual checkup to detect endometriosis early enough to treat it; have infections treated promptly, as they can cause tubal damage; use effective contraceptive techniques so you will not need an abortion, which can decrease a woman's reproductive efficiency. What's missing here—what's missing in most of what you read or are told about avoiding infertility problems—is a single word about the nutrition of the childless couple.

A veterinarian faced with an infertile cow doesn't talk to her about her IUD. He first checks the animal's diet and suggests improvements. An interesting thing about cattle is that one of the nutrition devices used to help the reproductive efficiency of animals is feeding them concentrated fractions of wheat. In human terms that translates into more vitamin B complex, unsaturated fatty acid, vitamin E, and a group of minerals.

It seems most of the medical establishment has never heard there's a relationship between one's previous diet and one's fertility. Yet I'm happy to say there are a considerable number of babies who were born to couples who had been infertile, who had gone through the usual medical procedures with no success, but who succeeded in conceiving when their diets were changed. One woman writes:

> Thirty-eight years ago, Dr. Fredericks, after three years
> of marriage I wrote to you about my inability to conceive.
> I had been an ardent listener of yours and your pre-con-
> ception diet worked so well that after receiving it in 1946,

I had a daughter in 1947, another in 1950, and then in 1955 I was pregnant with my third daughter.

The pre-pregnancy diet I sent her, which is to be used by both husband and wife prior to conception, I took from a diet tested at the University of Pennsylvania many years ago. It was tested on one thousand expectant mothers with a thousand controls on ordinary diets. In the group given the special diet the incidence of premature birth was dramatically reduced. I adapted this diet, adding things to make it useful for people who are having trouble conceiving.

There are hundreds of babies, many of them grown up, for whom I am the nutritional godfather. They were born to couples who could not conceive until their diets were changed. But, don't mistake me, we also have our failures. Again, the diet I'm talking about is for both the woman and the man. We're going beyond sperm counts and motility appraisal—the usual standards by which male fertility is measured.

The relationship of nutrition to pregnancy goes beyond allowing a malnourished woman to become pregnant and then trying to compensate during the months of pregnancy, with a double drain on her body, to make up for a long history of inadequate diet; of trying to compensate for the impact of morning sickness on nutrition; beyond the type of diet obstetricians have prescribed for their patients when they see edema or a rise in blood pressure—a low-calorie, low-protein, low-salt diet—to try to prevent toxemia and preeclampsia.

If I had my druthers I'd place both partners on a good diet for at least six months before conception is attempted. This isn't as radical as it sounds: There are some groups in the South Seas who will not permit a couple to attempt conception unless they've both been on a special diet for a significant period of time. Even with the best possible diet, I still want it supplemented intelligently.

105

Overcoming years of indifferent nutrition requires a more potent intake of some nutrients than food alone can supply.

I seldom see patients who come in looking for a good diet in pregnancy. I see childless couples who have gone through all the hormone therapies and other treatments, and are still unable to reproduce. Nothing can replace a complete physical examination and necessary corrective measures for both partners. But in corrective measures I do not include arbitrary dosing with hormones of various types. Even if it's successful in inducing conception, what service does hormone therapy perform if it allows conception in a poorly nourished mother by a poorly nourished father? The forces that affect the fetus do not operate in women alone, and they don't start operating only after conception has taken place. One cannot make promises that improved nutrition will create fertility in a barren marriage, but I can promise that neglecting proper nutrition is prejudicial not only to reproduction but to the welfare of the baby. There is no single magic factor in nutrition that stimulates fertility. Reproduction rests ultimately on all of the essential nutrients in a good diet.

If you went to the library and looked up the literature on human nutrition and reproduction you would find a report written about twenty-five years ago on the effect of a single nutrient, paraaminobenzoic acid (PABA), which was reported to help infertile women to conceive. The endocrinologist who investigated this effect of PABA never thought in terms of hormone deficiency alone or of nutritional deficiency alone. Rather, he investigated the impact of bad nutrition on hormone chemistry and the impact of disturbed hormone chemistry on nutritional utilization.

In this PABA investigation, twenty-two infertile women were given two hundred milligrams of PABA daily. Twelve of the women became pregnant and delivered successfully within two years. PABA is certainly no panacea, and certainly should not be employed until both parents have had a thorough medical exam. Nature sometimes blocks conception because the ovum or the sperm or both may be in some way abnormal, threatening miscarriage or, worse, the birth of a defective baby.

In the diet I recommend be used in pregnancy and to achieve conception, I am suggesting something that is not just the product of my fertile imagination; I am following guidelines that were thoroughly tested in a thousand pregnancies in tests run years ago at the University of Pennsylvania. In those cases the diet reduced premature births by a remarkable percentage. Premature birth is one of the great problems that raises medical insurance costs and inflicts a burden on government funds. More time spent on intensive care of the woman before she conceives will result in less need for intensive care of the premature infant.

The Pregnancy Diet

The following is the daily diet for mothers-to-be to use in the later months of pregnancy and during lactation. Fathers-to-be will find it a healthy diet, too.

Fruits

8 ounces freshly squeezed fruit juice, unstrained, preferably citrus

Commercially prepared fruit juices are not an acceptable substitution because they are often strained, and some of the vitamin C can be lost in the preparation and packaging. Unstrained, the juice will help protect you against varicose veins, which, if they develop, are treated with citrus bioflavonoids.

1 serving of fresh fruit, peeled

Ordinarily I wouldn't want the fruit to be peeled, but in pregnancy it is advisable to do so in order to minimize intake of pesticide

107

residue. Both fresh apples and apple juice should be avoided, unless your vegetable vendor or supermarket manager can assure you the apples have not been sprayed. You can substitute sweet potatoes and yams for apples in your diet.

Vegetables

2 cups of slightly undercooked vegetables (reserve cooking water)

Boil the cooking water down very rapidly in a shallow skillet. This destroys a minimum of the vegetable nutrients in the water and concentrates the rest. Use this as a stock when making gravies, or you can mix it with carrot juice.

1 cup of salad made with dark green leafy vegetables and olive oil with wheat germ oil dressing (season as desired)

Remember to thoroughly wash the salad greens and other vegetables to remove dirt and as much other residue as possible.

Oils and Fats

5 teaspoons or fewer of vegetable oil, plus 1 teaspoon of wheat germ oil

Olive oil is best; if you use other vegetable oils, don't use any that are hydrogenated or contain the petroleum-based preservatives BHA or BHT. You can add one tablespoon of wheat germ oil to the vegetable oil. Wheat germ oil has a specific action in helping reproduction. Keep all oils refrigerated and thoroughly sealed.

3 pats of butter

Do not use margarine. It contains partially hydrogenated fat, which isn't good for you or your baby-to-be.

Cereals

1 serving of oatmeal or other whole-grain cereal, to which
1 teaspoon of wheat germ and 1 tablespoon of coarse bran
should be added

Oatmeal, whole wheat, or any other whole-grain cereal is fine. The coarse bran should not always be wheat bran only; oat bran is also available. The bran helps elimination, but it will not help if you do not take sufficient liquids, including water. By the way, insufficient intake of fluid is a major cause of kidney stones.

Eggs, Meat, Fish

2 eggs

If you like to eat bacon with your eggs, be sure to find brands that do not contain nitrates or nitrites. These preservatives, which are often used in larger amounts than necessary so the meat products will have a pleasing color, are converted by heating and in the body into nitrosamines, which are extremely potent in causing cancer. If you do insist on eating bacon or other products when they do contain nitrates or nitrites take a small amount of vitamin C immediately after the meal to cancel the cancer-causing reaction.

6 ounces of red meat, fish, or fowl daily

We want an emphasis on organ meats. The price of liver is very low, yet nutritionally it is infinitely valuable. Fish in the diet is also important. You need an adequate intake of Omega 3 oils and the best source is the oily type of cold-water fish: salmon, mackerel, trout, sardines—there's a long list of fish of this type. On days when you do not eat fish, I suggest you take a teaspoonful of cod-liver oil—both partners! This may astonish you, but fish oil is important for the development of the baby's eyes. The fish should be particularly emphasized if the woman was taking birth-control pills prior to pregnancy. Fish oil is an antidote to the birth-control pills' blood-clotting action, which can be a cause of stroke.

Grains

> 4 slices of whole wheat, whole rye, or whole corn bread, or substitute servings of whole-grain pasta products

The rye does not mean commercial rye bread, which is simply a variation on white bread. Pumpernickel is merely commercial rye bread with an artificial suntan, namely caramel coloring. Make sure the bread you eat is whole-grain. Conventional spaghetti, macaroni, and noodles shouldn't be used. Use the high-protein pasta products. There are a number of these on the market with added soy flour and added wheat germ. Brewer's yeast, wheat germ, and nonfat dry skim milk should always be added to the appropriate recipes.

Desserts

> whole gelatin with fruit; yogurt; home-baked whole wheat cake, cookies, muffins

When you get to desserts don't take the attitude that here is where you can slip. Everything counts. Instead of buying commercial flavored gelatin desserts that consist of 15 percent gelatin, 85 percent sugar, artificial flavor, and artificial color, use whole gelatin and add stewed fruit or fruit whip. Use yogurt and learn how to make it at home. The prepared yogurt in stores is frequently messed up with a lot of added sugar, jams, and preserves. Make your own cakes, cookies, and muffins: Use whole grain as much as possible, and if you do use unbleached white flour add a teaspoon of whole wheat germ (not defatted wheat germ!) for each cup of flour.

I tend to be conservative about potencies of vitamin supplements used in pregnancy. I advise no more than 100 units of vitamin E (mixed tocopherols); approximately 250 milligrams of vitamin C in time-release form, which keeps the level up; not more than 50 micrograms of selenium. The supplements taken in the pre-conception period differ from those taken during pregnancy only by the extra PABA taken before conception.

Some of the supplementary foods you can use are bran and brewer's yeast. Use them as follows:

- BRAN: In addition to adding bran to your breakfast cereal, you can add it to yogurt, waffles, and pancakes (1 teaspoon of bran for each cup of flour)
- BREWER'S YEAST: Once pregnancy is confirmed, take 6 tablets daily, or substitute desiccated liver

If you are not eating fruit or unstrained fruit juice in the recommended amounts, you should take a supplement of one thousand milligrams of citrus bioflavonoids. I followed an experiment fifty years ago on the addition of bioflavonoids and vitamin C to the diets of pregnant women. Those in the experiment who took the supplements had a fraction of the varicose vein problems compared with those in the experiment who did not receive the supplements. An ounce of prevention!

Vitamin B$_6$ and Pregnancy

The fertility of both partners requires nutritional stimulation. If you don't follow this advice, don't be astonished if you run into

111

some of the things that are accepted, unfortunately, as "normal" consequences of pregnancy, as if pregnancy were a disease. For example, carpal tunnel syndrome, a disorder affecting the wrists and the hands, and that may also involve "trigger finger" and "tennis elbow." Victims of carpal tunnel syndrome suffer intense numbness, tingling, swelling, and chronic muscular weakness or atrophy. In long-standing cases there may be involvement of the shoulder, so the disorder is sometimes called shoulder/hand syndrome. The disorder is blamed on pressure on a nerve; however, thanks to the research of Dr. Carl Folker and Dr. John Alvis we have learned that deficiency in vitamin B_6 can cause this painful condition. Evidence for the role of this deficiency came from observing pregnant women who often have swelling of the hands and feet and often show clear evidence of carpal tunnel syndrome.

In pregnancy there appears to be interference with the metabolizing of vitamin B_6. That means there is a heightened requirement for it. The need often comes in the stage of pregnancy when morning sickness (itself often caused by lack of vitamin B_6) interferes with food intake. It is therefore not unexpected that vitamin B_6 would promptly relieve carpal tunnel syndrome in pregnant women. The same vitamin is used to treat one type of morning sickness.

Morning Sickness. Food cravings or aversions and nausea during the first three months of pregnancy are common worldwide. As far as nausea—morning sickness—is concerned, one of the theories involves vitamin B_6, a nutrient important in the detoxifying process. The normal detoxifying mechanism works during the night, when there is a great demand for vitamin B_6. But during pregnancy vitamin B_6 is needed as the placenta develops in the early months; because supplies of B_6 are being used in this way, and because too this nutrient is not found in many foods and tends to dissipate quickly, toxins in the system are not taken care of during the night and this is what makes the pregnant woman feel sick the next morning. There is another theory that in the first three months of pregnancy there is a physiological block on the utilization of vitamin B_6, which would have the same effect. Vitamin B_6 may also be related to aversion. Aversion is sometimes predicated on a distortion of the taste sense, which is easily created by zinc deficiency. Absorption of zinc is increased 40 percent by vitamin B_6.

Considering the birth-defects controversy that surrounds drugs used to control nausea in pregnancy, I strongly suggest acupressure techniques be tried for alleviating morning sickness. This is not an uncomplicated subject, as there appear to be three types of nausea in pregnancy. Vitamin B_6 is effective for one type—but is not effective in controlling the other types.

Newborns' Apgar Scores. A very strong relationship has been found between the amount of vitamin B_6 in a woman's diet during pregnancy and the Apgar score of her newborn. The Apgar score is a standard measure used to evaluate a baby's health immediately after birth. The Apgar score one minute after birth has been found to be higher for infants of women who took pyridoxine, vitamin B_6, during pregnancy than in infants of women who did not. Apparently the relationship between the woman's vitamin B_6 level and the baby's Apgar score is so strong that doctors are convinced that if more pregnant women had higher intake of vitamin B_6 we might have fewer babies who are in need of intensive care and other special steps, not only in order to keep life going, but in order to repair some of the organic or functional defects from which they suffer.

Suppressed Lactation. There is an action of B_6 I don't like to tell you about because I very much favor breast-feeding, but in women who don't want to breast-feed, vitamin B_6 is remarkably effective and safe in suppressing lactation. A British medical report based on studies of 254 women indicates that although vitamin B_6 works in a way that is still a mystery, it is much more effective and safer than estrogen in suppressing lactation. (Estrogen is the orthodox

113

medical treatment for milk suppression.) B$_6$ relieves the engorge-
ment of the breasts within ten to thirteen hours, which is half the
time taken for the estrogen treatment. It leads to complete suppression of milk formation within one week in more than 90 percent
of the women who take it and is trouble-free.

Maternal Folic Acid Deficiency

In a study of 805 women in early pregnancy, low levels of folic
acid were found in 135. Among the latter, the frequency of mal-
formation in their babies was four times greater than among the
670 women who had normal levels of the vitamin. You can add to
that a dozen other reports, including one in the *British Medical
Journal* on how folic acid was given to a group of women who had
delivered malformed babies in previous pregnancies, thus reducing
the incidence of deformity in the subsequent pregnancy. (Women
who have had one defective baby are more likely to have another.)
They gave folic acid to one group; they gave a placebo to the other
group. This means they brought defective babies into the world to
rule out the possibility that the power of suggestion could protect
an unborn baby from being deformed by a dietary deficiency. And
do you know the worst part of it? The work had already been done
five years before the British experiment and the results were clear-
cut: Folic acid cut down on defective births. Where is the moral
right, the ethical right to give a control group an empty capsule to
rule out the power of suggestion? And if the power of suggestion is
so darned effective, why does the American medical doctor consider
a faith healer a "quack"?

What bothers me most about these reports on malformed infants
is the emphasis on the woman. The father's diet prior to conception
also affects the baby because the father contributes genes; that point
has not been sufficiently stressed. It is the women who go to the
clinics for infertility; it is the women who go to the obstetricians

and seek help when in previous pregnancies they have had babies who were not normal. The husband likewise has a responsibility.

Let's trace folic acid as it goes through the body, because it has some unusual properties. It is not only a necessity in insuring the well-being of an adult's nervous system; it is also used to protect the health of the newborn. To find out why, take a look at the genes. The genes make us what we are and folic acid makes the genes what they are. Folic acid is very important to the formation of genes. Without the genes the blueprint is not there for the formation of organs. This explains the role of folic acid in preventing harelip, cleft palate, and spinal deformities in newborn babies. Here the gene has gone wrong because of lack of folic acid. The blueprint is not right; some instruction is being left out or distorted.

A scientist at the Massachusetts Institute of Technology has the theory that a marginal deficiency of folic acid in a mother-to-be might severely harm the child's ability to fight off disease later in life. In other words, the instructions from the genes to the immune system would be improperly transmitted. In laboratory tests using rats, the offspring of mothers fed diets with marginal amounts of folic acid were less able to overcome a type of bacteria that very commonly causes food poisoning than the offspring whose mothers received adequate amounts of folic acid. You would hardly think that your susceptibility to food poisoning would be related to your previous diet, but judging from the experiments, that is evidently the case.

Besides causing a greater chance of birth deformities or slower development in the child or impaired immune function, folic acid deficiency in the pregnant woman brings on toxemia of pregnancy, premature separation of the placenta from the wall of the uterus, and anemia.

The most marked symptom of folic acid deficiency is a type of anemia in which the red blood cells are too large. They are oddly shaped, and even though the normal life span of the red blood cell is short, these have a very short life span indeed. Moreover, in folic

115

acid deficiency the cells responsible for fighting infection also become excessively large and have a very short life span. They lose their ability to defend the body against viruses and bacteria. That inability is reversed if folic acid treatment is instituted.

This offers a possible answer to a question I very often receive. It goes something like this: I am very susceptible to every bug that comes through the population; I get every virus that comes along. Why? To which the answer is—and this is very frequently said of children, too—sometimes inadequate intake of vitamin C and folic acid can make you the happy hunting ground for viruses and bacteria.

Studies carried out by the World Health Organization would seem to contradict the impression that folic acid deficiency is confined only to poor women who don't eat properly. They estimate that aside from the United States, one-third of all the pregnant women in the world have folic acid deficiency. This is tragic because it becomes a vicious circle. Because the pregnant woman is herself more susceptible to infection, her child is more susceptible to prenatal influences that can cause deformity. The child, in turn, is later susceptible to infection. Many of these children live in areas where proper sanitation and medical care are not available. A test was done by Dr. Victor Herbert and several of his colleagues on 110 pregnant women who came from low-income families in New York City. Much to my astonishment, Dr. Herbert reported that one woman in six had a definite folic acid deficiency. (I say I was astonished because Dr. Herbert had pursued a long career of denigrating natural foods and decrying the use of vitamin supplements which, at least in this study, would have done his subjects some good.) Another 14 percent had a marginal folic acid deficiency. Thus a full 30 percent in the group were in trouble.

That study involved only women from a poor neighborhood. Dr. Charles A. Hall and his coworkers, associated with the nutrition program at the Albany Medical College, New York, tested the folate levels of 106 healthy women. They found that one in every three was on the edge of a folic acid deficiency. Remembering that this vitamin affects the genes, don't you have to wonder how many of those people were responsible for the conception of a baby during this period when their folic acid levels were low? To what extent was the baby compromised? How many babies were in some way defective?

Do you want to get a folic acid deficiency in a hurry? Very easy: Just take birth-control pills. A woman takes birth-control pills and so develops vitamin B_6 and folic acid deficiencies. When she decides to become pregnant and stops taking the pill what will happen to her baby? Birth defects are a real possibility. So when you decide to become pregnant, even before you stop the pill, put yourself on a program of good nutrition.

There is a large volume of research that indicates taking antibiotics can also cause folic acid deficiency. Folic acid is believed to be manufactured to some extent by bacteria in the digestive tract, and antibiotics kill off this friendly bacteria. This also needs to be taken into account if you are planning to become pregnant.

Caffeine and Pregnancy

Caffeine intake and the sugar people often add to coffee can become strongly addictive. There has been denial that caffeine causes any deformity of the unborn. I will note that this denial comes from the Harvard School of Nutrition and I have some reservation about the association between that school and a large number of industries. There is a study, however, that indicates that an intake of coffee in late pregnancy definitely carries hazards.

In the later stages of pregnancy, caffeine is not excreted from a woman's body. Compared with excretion of the drug during the final weeks of pregnancy, in two to twelve weeks after delivery the clearance of caffeine from the body increases by a factor of more than three. Before delivery the caffeine is retained, crosses the

117

placenta, and reaches the fetus. This is much the same as the situation with alcohol—if you wouldn't give your baby a cocktail, don't take one yourself. If a woman doesn't decrease her intake of coffee, tea, and other sources of caffeine in the late stages of pregnancy the concentration of caffeine in the fetus's blood will reach a level three times as high as the caffeine level in nonpregnant women drinking coffee. You're giving the fetus quite a dose in the later stages of pregnancy—I suggest that you don't.

Varicose Veins

Varicosities in pregnant women are often blamed on the extra weight they gain. Apparently, though, if we follow this line of reasoning, there are some pregnant women who don't bear extra weight! The husband carries it obviously. The pregnant women who are on high intake of vitamin C have one-tenth the amount of varicose veins as their counterparts who are on low intake of vitamin C. So there definitely is a dietary factor involved. This research was done by William Martin at the Women's Lying-in Hospital in Manhattan in 1939. I know. I was there. The study examined the incidence of varicose veins among the low-income pregnant women who came into the hospital clinic as compared to the incidence among the more affluent pregnant women he saw in his private practice. Dr. Martin found nine times as many cases of varicose veins among the lower-income women. He traced the cause to a diet providing inadequate amounts of vitamin C and bioflavonoids—the more affluent women could afford oranges.

Unnecessary Episiotomy During Childbirth

The episiotomy is an effort to prevent tearing of the perineum in childbirth by making an incision. However, it is more a con-

118

venience for the surgeon than a benefit for the woman. Where episiotomy was done only when medically necessary, the procedure was performed in 8 percent of the deliveries as compared to the usual 89 percent. So if there is a medical reason, fine, but in most deliveries an episiotomy is not necessary yet it is performed anyway. I have seen cases where a muscle was damaged by this procedure, a risk that is usually totally uncalled for. When obstetricians get used to their patients delivering in a birthing chair rather than in the supine position on the delivery table, the episiotomy will probably begin to disappear except in those few cases where there is some sort of pathology. The same goes for enemas before delivery. They were done routinely in the United States for many years. This arbitrary practice has been dropped in many other countries and is beginning to fall off here, too.

Breast-Feeding versus Bottle-Feeding

There is only one food on the face of the earth to which we can point with certainty and say, "This was intended for consumption by humans." That food is human breast milk. Yet, what have we done? We have substituted cow's milk—boiled, diluted, modified with cornstarch or corn syrup or sugar or lactose or whatever—to nurture our infants. In so doing we left behind the immune factors the mother passes on to her baby via breast milk.

For many years we have recognized that breast milk is the best invention for feeding a child; that no cunning of chemists or manufacturers has improved on the product of the mammary glands. At the same time we are aware that the mother's diet must be good: A malnourished mother is not going to produce high-quality milk. In fact this is the reason for the suggestion made by the group who have been having a battle with the Nestlé corporation.

Nestlé, along with other organizations, was selling infant formulas in developing nations to mothers who might be better off nursing

119

their babies. They went to mothers in areas where the cash income is less than one hundred dollars a year with a costly substitute for breast milk that is not equal to breast milk and never will be. Given the high cost of the formula, many believe that the mothers diluted it excessively to make it last, and this may have contributed to the incidence of deficiency diseases. Based on these allegations, the World Health Organization was called in and people began boycotting Nestlé and its subsidiary companies. One woman made the wonderful suggestion that the formulas be labeled "Milk Improver" and sold to nursing mothers for their own use, while they continued to nurse their babies.

Many of you have probably heard that breast-fed babies have colic less frequently than formula-fed babies. That's very true. Cow's milk causes havoc with infants' digestion. If a nursing mother is drinking cow's milk, she may absorb unaltered protein molecules from the cow's milk and transmit them to her infant in her breast milk. The infant's intestinal tract is not selective at that stage. The whole chain of allergies often starts with the infants' absorption of unaltered cow's-milk proteins.

It has long been known that some substances can pass from mother to infant in breast milk and cause adverse reactions. In one study on the relationship between colic and the nursing mother's consumption of cow's milk, colic disappeared in thirty-five of sixty-six breast-fed infants whose mothers were put on diets free of cow's milk. When twenty-three of the mothers again added cow's milk to their diets, on at least two occasions colic reappeared. There are contradictory reports in the literature, but this may be because soy milk products are often substituted for cow's milk in such studies and soy milk may also cause colic. It appears that in one-third of breast-fed infants with colic, the problem may be solved by removing cow's milk from the mother's diet.

There really isn't any substitute for breast-feeding, regardless of the grandiloquent claims of the formula manufacturers. Over the years, formulas were sadly deficient in important nutrients, the lack of which was not recognized except in hindsight. I recall one baby who was severely brain-damaged for life as a result of being fed a formula that was advertised as "the nearest thing to mother's milk" and that turned out not to be an adequate source of vitamin B_6. Human breast milk contains turine and *Lactobacillus bifidus* and neither of these is found in cow's milk, from which most infant formulas are made. Turine is an amino acid that acts as a regulator of the brain and nervous system. The absence of *Lactobacillus bifidus* in infant formula is thought to be a major reason why formula-fed infants have more gastrointestinal disorders than breast-fed infants.

Let me now give you the example of manganese. Infant formulas can contain three to one hundred times as much manganese as human milk. A study of breast-fed versus formula-fed infants found the manganese levels of the formula-fed infants declined from birth levels very slowly as compared to those of the breast-fed infants. Studies have shown that nursing animals absorb manganese more readily than mature animals and are more susceptible to manganese toxicity. In human adults manganese toxicity due to occupational exposure causes nervousness, irritability, compulsive behavior, emotional instability, and other symptoms, possibly due to damage to the neurons in the brain caused by manganese. Learning disabled children who are hyperactive and have short attention spans were found to have manganese levels in their hair 62 percent higher than normal children at ages seven to ten.

The substitution of the bottle for the breast may cause a narrow palate in a baby. Not only does the bottle not provide the kind of support for the mouth that the baby's palate needs, but if the aperture in the nipple is enlarged too much the baby may be faced with a flood of milk and will push the tongue forward in a thrusting motion that can contribute to distortion of the palate.

7
MENOPAUSE AND POSTMENOPAUSAL PROBLEMS

Sweats and Flushes

With the onset of menopause a woman's body produces less estrogen. This decreasing estrogen level is thought to be responsible for menopause symptoms—particularly the basal motor disturbances, the sweats and flushes—and for two other concerns of the postmenopausal woman, osteoporosis and atrophic vaginitis. The doctors say that as you go into menopause the estrogen level goes down and that's why you have sweats and flushes. But as I said earlier, if too little estrogen causes sweats and flushes, why don't ten-year-old girls who are low in estrogen have sweats and flushes? Why don't men have them? In one double-blind, carefully controlled study, with estrogen measured against a placebo, the sweats and flushes of those who took the placebo were more successfully controlled than in those who took the estrogen.

There's been a swing back to using estrogen replacement therapy for treating menopausal symptoms. Estrogen and progesterone are given in a cycle. The gynecologists and others who use estrogen in treating the menopause defend themselves by saying they are giving it with the so-called antidotal hormone, progesterone. If you must use estrogen, you can ensure safe progesterone production with vitamin B_6. Vitamin B complex in the diet is a critical factor in controlling estrogen, whether it is prescribed by a doctor or produced by the ovaries.

In an orthodox medical office women often end up with a tranquilizer for treatment of menopausal symptoms. In the nutritionist's office, we make an attempt to correct the chemistry and counterbalance the effects of estrogen. As far as the flushes go, vitamin E, ginseng tea, and riboflavonoids will provide relief.

Vitamin E is used for the treatment of menopausal flushing. It has an antithyroid effect, and a flush starts in the thyroid. Normally there is a balance between estrogen and thyroid hormone; they complement each other. Underactivity of the thyroid has been identified with premenstrual syndrome and difficulties in the menstrual cycle, as has red blood cell deficiency.

Atrophic Vaginitis

Atrophic vaginitis is the drying of the vaginal tissue that occurs after menopause. It's very torturous for the patient because it makes intercourse very difficult. If you go to a gynecologist or a dermatologist you're going to end up with an estrogen cream; Cynomal or Premarin vaginal cream are often prescribed. Both have side effects and may also irritate you. What concerns me is that the estrogen does work for many women, but a dose of estrogen in a vaginal cream is exactly equivalent to a dose of estrogen by mouth.

Vitamin E cream has been a successful substitute for estrogen cream in a large number of women with atrophic vaginitis. The problem is finding one that is not perfumed; you're not looking for the additional problem of an allergic reaction. One company puts out a vitamin E suppository that would be worth looking for.

I think the combination of vitamin A cream with vitamin E

cream would make sense, and I've suggested to many physicians that when they prescribe this they have the patient open up some vitamin E capsules and stir the contents directly into the cream because the potency of a cream is very frequently not high enough. This relieves about 50 percent of the cases, which is a pretty good batting average.

There happens to be documentation in the literature on the action of vitamin E ointment in treating atrophic vaginitis. The attitude of those doctors who won't look into the use of vitamin E ointment for this painful problem is completely unforgivable. We are not dealing here with tissue which, if damaged, can never be repaired, and in addition this is a harmless vitamin. Women should be reluctant to use a cream containing estrogen, a dangerous hormone, and apply it to delicate vaginal tissue, where it can be absorbed.

Osteoporosis

You can't talk to me about needing estrogen therapy in menopause to reduce the risk of osteoporosis (weakening of the bones) because I will deal with it nutritionally. You can protect the skeleton with adequate intake of cod-liver oil (vitamin D) and calcium. But this needs to be done long before menopause, since it is always easier to prevent a disease than to treat one. I would start that prevention twenty years before osteoporosis might begin. With adequate intake of calcium and cod-liver oil, I anticipate that when a woman arrives at the age when osteoporosis becomes a hazard, it will not occur. That to me is a heck of a lot better than dosages of hormones whose safety is highly questionable.

Women who have an intake of one thousand to fifteen hundred milligrams of calcium a day are much less likely to get osteoporosis. You also must have an adequate amount of vitamin D—about 400 units a day. We have been supplementing women's diets with cal-

125

cium oratate preventively because it is very well absorbed, better than other forms of calcium, and we have also been giving vitamins A and D in the form of cod-liver oil. If you don't like the taste of cod-liver oil, capsules are available. I prefer the oil because there are other things in it not found in the capsules, including something that helps to prevent hardening of the arteries.

If you use calcium oratate as a supplement you don't need as large a dose as when you use dicalcium phosphate or calcium glutamate. Generally speaking, as a supplement I suggest five hundred milligrams of calcium oratate three times a day. For me this represents the kind of protection I'd like to see well before the menopause and certainly afterward.

8
OTHER NUTRITIONAL CONCERNS OF WOMEN

Birth-Control Pills

Many years ago I journeyed to Cincinnati to debate a premise to which I took violent exception: that the birth-control pill was safe. One of the palpable dangers is that the pill puts women into a state of simulated pregnancy for years, and no one can make a prediction of what happens when you create such a state. Beyond that there is a tacit admission of danger: We are told when you reduce the dose you reduce the danger of blood clots, heart attack, and stroke. If there wasn't any danger in the first place, why reduce the dose to lessen the danger?

Blood clots, heart attack, stroke: This is a roundup of the hazards of the birth-control pill and they are largely the hazards of estrogen, which I've already described. I remind you: Control of estrogen is a nutritional process. Long-term pill users have up to triple the risk of heart attack. The number of pill users at high risk of developing blood clots is about 6 percent.

Certainly in this turbulent world there are many things that can cause depression, from your own personal problems to what you read on the front pages of the newspaper. But there are some cases where you inflict depression on yourself. It has been recognized that birth-control pills can cause derangement of vitamin chemistry and as a result may cause psychological upset. I first brought that information to you in the third year the birth-control pills were on the market. Since that time the research papers have come out one after another: The pills interfere with folic acid metabolism; they lower vitamin C; they lower vitamin A; they interfere with vitamin B_6—there's a whole list of things they do, none of them desirable. According to some reports, as many as 34 percent of users of the pill show mild to moderate depression plus irritability, emotional lability, lethargy, and fatigue. Some of them develop paranoid ideas, because of the effect on vitamin B_6 metabolism, and 75 percent of the women with psychological upsets associated with the pill are helped by vitamin B_6. It is thought that B_6 induces the production of progesterone, the so-called antidote for estrogen. Antidotes for estrogen should be received cheerfully because that hormone can be responsible for so many troubles. If vitamin B_6 is responsible for progesterone production following the rise in estrogen production prior to menstruation, that is tantamount to saying that the vitamin is necessary for ovulation. For this reason B_6 can sometimes be the answer to a woman's infertility.

Folic Acid Deficiency

I told you earlier about folic acid deficiency that can happen when women take the birth-control pill. A woman takes the birth-control pill, she develops vitamin B_6 deficiency and then folic acid deficiency. When she stops taking the pill in order to become pregnant, she should be aware the pill caused these deficiencies and, even before she stops taking it, put herself on a program of good nutrition. If she doesn't, both she and her baby will suffer.

And I've mentioned the research that indicates that taking an-

128

tibiotics can cause a folic acid deficiency because antibiotics kill the friendly bacteria believed to manufacture folic acid to some extent, along with the unfriendly bacteria it's intended for.

Ninety percent of all alcoholics are deficient in folic acid, which means it would be more appropriate to serve spinach than coffee and donuts at meetings of alcoholics.

Folic Acid in Foods. Eat raw foods, not cooked ones. Foods boiled for fifteen minutes lose up to 80 percent of their folic acid. Romaine lettuce, spinach, parsley, and collard greens all have good amounts of folate. If you do cook the greens, I suggest the Chinese method. Cut them into shreds, heat a very small amount of vegetable oil in a wok or skillet, cook quickly while stirring until tender, no more than three to four minutes.

Wheat germ has a very good supply of folic acid and this is one of the reasons for using it to reinforce your cereal and to use it in recipes when you bake. Liver supplies ample amounts of folic acid; desiccated liver is a rich source. Brewer's yeast is perhaps the richest source of folic acid. It has three times more folic acid than a cup of raw spinach. Brewer's yeast can be added to soup, stew, chopped meat preparations, and baked goods. Caution: If you have candidiasis, don't use brewer's yeast as your source of folic acid.

Vitamin B_6

An application of vitamin B_6 that has become very important to women is its action in offsetting the negative effects of the birth-control pill. The oral contraceptives very often cause derangement of vitamin metabolism and as a result of this, there may be psychological disturbances as well. As I said earlier, vitamin B_6 metabolism is involved, and investigators have been reporting that in as many as three women out of four with psychological upsets associated with the pill, fifty milligrams of vitamin B_6 daily produced

129

marked improvement. Vitamin B_6 has also been helpful for women in offsetting the tendency to store water, particularly in the premenstrual week, and helps clear up premenstrual acne.

When you give vitamin B_6 to menstruating women in the premenstrual week, or start a little earlier at ovulation, there is an enormously beneficial effect on such symptoms as fluid retention, cramps, and anxiety.

Many other conditions are alleviated by vitamin B_6, including:

arthritis	neuritis	carpal tunnel syndrome
schizophrenia	anemia	autism
breath holding	hangover	hardening of the arteries
heart disease	stroke	morning sickness

On pages 43–44, I have told you about the doses of vitamin B_6 I recommend and something about food sources for it. But there's more that must be said.

Some provision was made for enrichment of flour and bread with vitamin B_6 but nothing was ever done to carry this out. Vitamin B_6, pantothenic acid, and vitamin E are still discarded during milling and still not restored.

Shredded wheat is represented as whole wheat; it has lost 37 percent of its vitamin B_6 content (which was in the original wheat). Cracked wheat bread has lost 48 percent of its vitamin B_6; puffed wheat, 56 percent. Puffed wheat antagonizes me for another reason as well. They weren't satisfied with the overprocessing, so they put the wheat into guns and explode it. That takes care of denaturing the protein, so the protein value goes down as does the vitamin B_6. Saltine crackers have lost 62 percent of their vitamin B_6; spaghetti, 64 percent; French bread, 70 percent; white bread, 77 percent; all-purpose flour, 82 percent; cake flour, 86 percent. Quantities up to 90 percent of the vitamin B_6 are removed from many popular foods.

From that list of foods and the amount lost in processing, it is obvious we need to take some precautions.

Chronic Indigestion

The greatest single cause of indigestion in my experience is excessive consumption of sugar. People who have been heavy sugar eaters all their lives are often those who have had indigestion all their lives and have been taking antacids and other indigestion remedies all their lives. Relief from indigestion can usually be brought about with a low-carbohydrate (low-sugar) diet. A large percentage of patients with chronic indigestion who have tried the low-carbohydrate diet not only report improvement, but some of them say they will never go off the diet after their experience with it. In one study, out of a group of thirty-nine patients, eleven showed no improvement in their indigestion on the low-carbohydrate diet, while twenty-eight found it was greatly relieved. In addition to chronic indigestion, digestive problems of members of the test group included gastric ulcer, duodenal ulcer, and hiatal hernia.

Sugar affects the walls of the stomach; they become red, irritated, inflamed. This is followed by an increase in the production of stomach acid. That increase in acid production will only mean trouble, especially for someone who already has an ulcer or hiatal hernia.

Varicose Veins

One in ten of us has varicose veins. There is a genetic factor— a genetic tendency to those ugly, swollen, knobby veins in the legs. It seems to run in families, as do poor dietary habits.

What happens when you have varicosities? If they're uncomplicated, bandages are used or specially fitted elastic stockings, which essentially are substituting for muscle or for muscle tone to facilitate the flow of blood. The fit is very critical on these stockings and the main drawback is that they stretch after a while and then don't offer the necessary support anymore. If that doesn't help sufficiently, a treatment called sclerotherapy is used, which involves injecting a chemical into the vein to destroy it. That is not as popular as it used to be, first because it fails frequently (it leaves brown pigment stains on the skin) and sometimes there are serious side effects. In addition, it is obviously symptomatic treatment. You're removing the malfunctioning vein, which is the evidence of the problem; you haven't done anything about the problem. Complete surgical removal of the vein is regarded today as the best approach when the varicosities are very significant. The most common method involves tying off the veins and removing them—it's also called stripping. The assumption is that once the defective vessels are removed, then the healthy ones will resume their function. But that, in my experience, is not what happens. What happens is the condition redevelops in the veins which were healthy, indicating, of course, that the underlying problem is still present. The nutritional approach is to raise your intake of vitamin E. Adequate intake of vitamin C and the bioflavonoids can also prevent varicose veins. Pregnant women with a high intake of vitamin C have one-tenth as many varicose veins as those who have a low intake of vitamin C.

Herpes

There are two main groups of viruses, one made up of DNA, the other of RNA. Many of the viruses that affect the skin are from the RNA group. This includes the viruses that cause genital warts and genital herpes, cold sores, and shingles. Viruses have a nasty habit. They enter a cell and change its chemistry so that the cell then produces the virus. For this reason they are hard to cure.

The herpes virus seems to migrate to the skin from the nerve cells, where it lives. Lysine, used to treat herpes, has had a lot of publicity because it is an antagonist to arginine, another amino acid, which the herpes virus happens to need. By blocking arginine, the lysine permits the virus to languish. It doesn't have the opportunity to reproduce itself because the arginine is necessary for that. Lysine has therefore been used to shorten herpes attacks and make them less severe. Large doses of lysine to block arginine can cause arginine deficiency, which causes sterility in males. Herpes attacks can also be shortened and made less severe with vitamin C in large amounts and with vitamin E. Vitamin B_{12} is also given orally or by injection to help diminish the severity of the attack, and B_{12} may also be helpful if applied locally.

There seems to be a good deal of the amino acid arginine in many foods of the nut family. Arginine is a protein needed by the herpes virus. As a result of that unhappy faculty, nuts are capable of causing cold sores. So those of you who find that at holiday times or other times when there are lots of nuts around you are prone to cold sores now know how an outbreak might be avoided! If you don't want to totally avoid nuts you should increase your intake of lysine.

Viral infections of the skin cause problems in two ways. The virus multiplies in the skin cells, damaging and sometimes killing the cells. The multiplication of the virus causes release of arachadonic acid, a fatty acid, from the cell membrane, where it's normally held in an inactive form. Once freed from the membrane the acid is converted to inflammatory products. The virus brings out of the cell something that is turned into a prostaglandin and that is extremely inflammatory.

As a result of research in several countries—the United States, Canada, Great Britain, and Sweden—an ointment to treat genital herpes has been developed. Lithium suxanate does not cross the skin so it does not get into the bloodstream and no cellular damage occurs.

Lithium can block the release of arachadonic acid and consequently prevents the formation of all the products the body makes from arachadonic acid, including the inflammatory and irritating forms of prostaglandins. The arachadonic acid remains in its inactive form. Lithium ions also have a unique action in blocking the RNA viruses from multiplying and yet does not hurt the cell in which the virus has taken up residence. Lithium ions do not interfere with DNA virus multiplication and so are highly specific in their action.

Lithium very rapidly relieves the pain and inflammation of viral skin infections—within one to two hours of being applied locally to the lesions. Because it blocks multiplication of the virus, if it is applied every four hours it will allow full healing of the lesions in one to three days, as compared to the six to eight days it would take if left untreated. Lithium suxanate is the form that gives the best results. It is available over-the-counter in health food stores.

Zinc's action is similar to that of lithium. It stimulates the formation of prostaglandin E-1, which is an antagonist of the prostaglandin that causes the inflammation. Zinc ions may also have a direct antiviral action, and zinc throat sprays are now being used for the type of sore throat that sometimes pops up with a viral infection. PEG-1 also has a lithium-like action in blocking the mobilization of the arachadonic acid released by the virus. Vitamin E inhibits one of the enzymes involved in inflammation caused by a virus and potentiates the anti-inflammatory effect of lithium.

A cream containing lithium suxanate, zinc sulfate, and vitamin E is probably the best choice for the control of viral infections of the skin. Used for genital herpes, cold sores, or shingles, this cream brought relief from pain within one to two hours and healing within one to three days. Applied to genital warts, it causes them to disappear in two to three weeks.

Both shingles and recurrent herpes infections are preceded by a prodromal period of several hours when the skin feels tingly and

134

itchy. Lithium suxanate ointment applied to the skin during this period can completely prevent the development of lesions, but you must reach the infection before it becomes fully active if you want that kind of prevention. Because all inflammatory infections of the skin are associated with the release of arachadonic acid, lithium suxanate can also be used effectively for contact dermatitis, eczema, and sunburn.

Anorexia Nervosa

I've never seen an anorexic who did not also have hypoglycemia, and very frequently because of the problem of getting these people to eat, the hypoglycemia is neglected. I have resorted to the use of a protein concentrate in powder form administered at two-hour intervals as a beverage. There are two reasons for that. The first is to overcome the problem that the person doesn't eat frequently enough, the second is that I've met with more success with underweight people and especially those with anorexia nervosa if I give something in liquid rather than chewable form. This has been quite helpful to some, but there is an underlying emotional problem involved in anorexia. I'd prefer a clinical psychologist, rather than a psychiatrist, be involved in treatment. I don't like some of the drugs that are prescribed, and because a clinical psychologist is not allowed to prescribe drugs their negative effects are avoided. Zinc has been found to be an almost routine deficiency in anorexics and they profit by its administration.

One treatment for anorexia nervosa involves bringing down the level of cortisone production in the body. When you suppress the corticosteroids, the adrenal hormones, you are not only affecting the anorexia, but also the entire body. This treatment should be attempted only on a short-term basis. It is not the entire solution to anorexia nervosa; there is still the emotional component.

Panic Attacks

Women are very often the sufferers of panic attacks. They usually end up on the psychiatrist's couch or take antianxiety drugs administered by a physician. Those drugs alter the chemistry of the brain and are to be avoided. But when a nutritionist alters the chemistry of the brain by using harmless nutrients, the orthodox medical community is up in arms about such quackery and faddism.

Hypoglycemia is a principal cause of these attacks. I have known of panic attacks totally ceasing once the sufferer is on a diet to combat low blood sugar. Caffeine contributes to hypoglycemia in some people and so is also tied to panic attacks. Caffeine may actually trigger panic attacks in some people, and hypoglycemia certainly does in a large number of people. The mind affects the body, and then there are the times when the body affects the mind.

9 | DIET PLANS FOR CONTROLLING ESTROGEN

What do you do about menu planning? If you do what the average consumer does in the U.S. today, you select food because it's on sale; because it comes in a pretty, reusable container; because you have a coupon this week that will save you money; because it's seasonally available; because you always serve pheasant and caviar on Thursday night; and so on. What's missing? Selecting foods that meet your nutritional needs. At that point menu planning is no longer simple.

I do not believe three meals a day make any sense. With three meals a day, when I look at your blood sugar, you go from starvation to plenty to starvation to plenty, and the curve goes up and down all day long. That is not the way to keep the body functioning properly. When you eat large meals, you stir up your enzyme system (if you don't, you're in trouble) and the enzyme system becomes very efficient in extracting from the food the maximum that can be extracted. When you eat small meals the enzyme system does not become agitated in that way. This adds up to a recommendation many of you may not be able to follow: Eat six meals a day instead of three—but take in the same amount of food. Despite the fact that it is the same amount of food, because of the change in enzyme action you will wind up with better weight control, lower cholesterol, and lower triglycerides (it is best not to have these abnormally high). You will also wind up feeling better fed and more efficient. The beneficial effect of this is profound to a degree that I don't think the average person recognizes.

The second thing vis-à-vis your menu planning most of you will balk at is to turn your day around and take your dinner at breakfast. I know this sounds revolting to those of you who stagger out of bed bleary-eyed, feeling entirely incapable of facing the world. Nevertheless, there are people who suffer from tiredness and swollen ankles, whose condition cannot be diagnosed or treated, but who improve if they are persuaded to take dinner at breakfast time! It is very difficult to change dietary habits. I've been trying it for half a century. It is almost impossible to get people to change the pattern of their meals until they have a compelling reason to do so.

The Basic Diet

The following list gives you the basic daily food framework for control of estrogen and good health. How many meals you divide this into is your choice. Some people feel and function better on frequent small meals (which do make weight control easier), others simply can't eat more than two meals daily, and there are those who function on one meal, though it's difficult to achieve a balanced diet when it rests on only one leg. The pattern of three meals a day is simply a concession to the schedules of bus, job, or school and has no relationship to the body's actual needs.

- fruit juice, unstrained, 1 8-ounce glass. Preferably citrus; fresh-squeezed is superior to canned or frozen.
- fresh fruit, unpeeled, 1 serving. Wash thoroughly.

- vegetables, cooked, 2 cups. Choose from as wide a variety as possible. Serve slightly undercooked.
- salad, 1 cup. Use dark green leafy vegetables. Dressing should be pure vegetable oils; season as you prefer.
- butter, 3 squares.
- oatmeal, whole wheat, or other cereal, 1 serving. Whole-grain with 1 teaspoon of defatted wheat germ added and whole or nonfat milk. Whole-grain pancakes or waffles may be substituted. A teaspoon or two of coarse miller's bran in the cereal will help to keep elimination normal.
- eggs, 2 daily. Cooked in any style or used in eggnogs, baked dishes, custards, etc.
- lean meat, fish, fowl, or cheese, 6 ounces. Individually or in any combination. Meat selections should emphasize organs—liver, kidney, tripe, sweetbreads.
- stone-ground whole-grain bread, 4 slices. Whole wheat, whole rye, or whole corn. Whole-grain pasta products may be substituted. Do not use conventional spaghetti, macaroni, and noodles.
- milk, 3 glasses. The equivalent in cheese, buttermilk, kefir, or yogurt may be substituted, or recipes in which milk is a significant ingredient.
- brewer's yeast, wheat germ, and nonfat dried milk can be added to appropriate recipes.
- Desserts: nutritious whole-grain, low-sugar cookies or cakes; whole gelatin, junket, or custard with fruit; stewed or fresh fruit with or without cheese; fruit whip. No convenience desserts, commercial cakes, cookies, or ice cream (it's 16 percent sugar and may have additives) or whipped toppings. Use real cream. Some excellent whole-grain cookies and cakes are available in health food stores.
- Snacks: nuts and seeds within your calorie limitations. These are sources of new life and filled with the nutrients needed to support it. If you are a snacker, these choices concentrate

your good nutrition rather than dilute it as ordinary snacks do.

Food Sensitivities. In the Basic Diet there are a dozen possible impasses for the food-sensitive, including those with allergies or intolerances to whole grains, bran, wheat germ, milk, cheese, uncooked fruit, salad greens, organ meats, or even brewer's yeast. And there are a small number of people who won't be able to use some of the supplements (see chapter 10) that can compensate for restrictions on food selection. Here are some ideas to help those who must find alternatives to some of the good foods in the Basic Diet.

- CITRUS FRUITS. If these don't agree with you use those fruits and juices you do find friendly. Tomato juice is good—it is lower in vitamin C than citrus, but the deficit can be made up for in supplements. Apple juice fortified with vitamin C is useful, though its high carbohydrate content would be a problem for those who function best on a low-carbohydrate diet. Pineapple juice is another possible choice, but one with too much sugar to make calorie watchers happy.
- RAW VEGETABLES AND SALAD GREENS. If you are intolerant of these, some of the cooked vegetables may also cause you a problem. Pureed vegetables and vegetable juices will partially compensate.
- WHOLE GRAINS. You can achieve some of their essential values by fortifying processed cereals and unbleached white flour with wheat germ, starting with one teaspoonful per cup and gradually increasing when tolerance is established.
- MILK AND CHEESE. Allergy is the usual reason milk disturbs people, but the reaction may also be due to lack of an enzyme needed to break down lactose. If you compulsively crave milk, allergy is the problem. Those with the problem of the missing enzyme can try the lactose-reduced milk now on the market; some can tolerate fermented milk products, such as

kefir, yogurt, or acidophilus milk. Occasionally certified raw milk is better accepted than pasteurized milk. Some people are able to drink ordinary pasteurized milk if it has been brought to a boil and then quickly cooled. Those intolerant of naturally ripened cheeses made from pasteurized milk may have less difficulty with cheeses from Switzerland, where the milk used is not pasteurized. Dairy products have a high-quality protein value and contain a rich store of vitamins and minerals, particularly calcium. If, however, you can't consume them, your supplements will protect you.

The Reducing Diet

To eat well you need three thousand calories a day of well-selected foods. The Basic Diet was created with a reasonable consideration of the calorie ceiling women generally wish to observe, but it is obviously not aimed at those who must lose weight. The following diet is a tested, highly successful, well-balanced reducing diet arranged so you needn't count calories and can stay within your diet even when dining away from home. If you are in normal health and your metabolism is normal this diet should melt away about two pounds per week, which is about as fast a weight loss as anyone should try to achieve.

BREAKFAST

1 serving of fruit
1 egg or egg substitute
½ slice (thin) whole-wheat toast with ½ level tsp. butter
1 glass of skim milk
1 cup of coffee or tea (optional), with no sugar, cream, or milk

141

LUNCH

1 helping of lean meat, fish, fowl, or meat substitute
1 vegetable from Vegetable List A
1 salad (from Salad List)
1 serving of fruit or dessert
1 glass of skim milk or buttermilk
1 cup of coffee or tea (optional), with no sugar, cream, or milk

DINNER

1 cup of soup (optional)
1 helping of lean meat, fish, fowl, or meat substitute
2 vegetables from Vegetable List A and 1 from Vegetable List B

or

1 vegetable from Vegetable List A plus 1 from Vegetable List B
    plus 1 helping of salad (from Salad List)
1 portion of fruit or dessert
Coffee or tea (no sugar, cream, or milk)

Choose foods from the following lists:

SOUP LIST

Consommé
Clear vegetable soup
Beef broth
Mutton broth
Chicken broth
Other clear soups
NOTE: No creamed soups, none with milk or content of vegetables,
    meat, or cereals.

FRUIT LIST

Orange (1, small)
Grapefruit (½, medium size)
Apple, (1, small)
Pineapple (2 average slices)
Peach (1)
Cantaloupe (½, medium size)
Melon (2-inch section of average-size melon)
Tangerine (1, large)
Berries (½ cup)
Apricots (2, medium size)
Grapes (12)
Cherries (10)
Pear (1, medium size)
Plums (2)
Nectarines (3)
Persimmon (½, small)
Fruit juices: 6 ounces (¾ water glass) grapefruit, orange (unsweetened)

MEAT LIST

Lean beefsteak (¼ lb., about 1 in. thick, 2½ in. square)
Roast beef (2 slices, about 3 in. square, ¼ in. thick)
Beef liver (1 slice, 3 in. square, ½ in. thick)
Beef tongue (2 average slices)
Beef kidney (¼ lb.)
Hamburger (¼ lb.)
Calf's liver (¼ lb.)
Lamb kidney (2, average size)
Lamb chop (1, about 2 in. square, ½ in. thick)
Roast lamb (1 slice, 3½ in. square, ¼ in. thick)
Mutton chop (2, medium size)

143

Boiled mutton (1 slice, 4 in. square, ½ in. thick)
Roast veal (1 slice, 3 in. by 2 in., ¼ in. thick)
Veal cutlet (1, average size)
Veal kidney (2, average size)
Chicken, white meat (2 slices, 4 in. square, cut very
    thin)
Chicken, broiler (½, medium size)
Chicken gizzards (2, average size)
Chicken livers (2 whole, medium size)

FISH LIST

Sea bass (¼ lb.)
Bluefish (¼ lb.)
Cod, fresh (¼ lb. to ½ lb.)
Cod, salt (¼ lb. to ½ lb.)
Flounder (¼ lb. to ½ lb.)
Haddock (¼ lb. to ½ lb.)
Halibut (¼ lb.)
Kingfish (¼ lb.)
Pike (¼ lb.)
Porgy (¼ lb.)
Red snapper (¼ lb.)
Scallops (⅔ cup, raw measurement)
Shrimp (⅔ cup)
Smelt (¼ lb.)
Weakfish (¼ lb.)
Clams, round (10 to 12)
Crab meat (1 crab or ¾ cup flakes)
Lobster (½ small lobster or 1 cup flakes)
Mussels (4 large or 8 small)
Oysters (12 large)

MEAT SUBSTITUTES

Cottage cheese (²/₃ cup)
Eggs (2)
Buttermilk (2 cups)
Whole milk (1 cup)
Skim milk (2 cups)

EGGS

Plain omelet
Poached
Soft-boiled
Hard-boiled
Raw

SUBSTITUTES FOR ONE EGG

Cottage cheese (4 Tbs.)
Lamb chop (1 small, lean)
Lamb kidney (1)
Calf's liver (2 oz.)
Mutton chop (1 small, lean)
Buttermilk (1 glass)
Skim milk (1 glass)

VEGETABLE LIST A

Asparagus (fresh or canned: 8)
String beans (½ cup)
Wax beans (½ cup)
Beet greens (2 heaping Tbs.)
Broccoli (1 5-in. stalk)
Brussels sprouts (½ cup)

145

Cabbage, cooked (½ cup)
Cabbage, raw (¾ cup, shredded)
Cauliflower (½ cup)
Celery (5 stalks)
Chard (½ cup)
Chicory (½ cup)
Eggplant (½ cup)
Endive (10 medium stalks)
Green pepper (1, medium size)
Kohlrabi (2 heaping Tbs.)
Leeks, chopped (⅓ cup)
Lettuce (10 leaves)
Radishes (5, medium size)
Sauerkraut (½ cup)
Spinach (½ cup)
Tomatoes, fresh (1)
Tomatoes, canned (½ cup)
Tomato juice: four ounces (½ cup)
Watercress (10 pieces)

VEGETABLE LIST B

Beets (2 heaping Tbs.)
Carrots (2 heaping Tbs.)
Chives (6)
Dandelion greens (3 heaping Tbs.)
Kale (2 heaping Tbs.)
Onion (2, small size)
Parsnips (2 heaping Tbs.)
Peas (2 heaping Tbs.)
Pumpkin (3 heaping Tbs.)
Rutabaga (2 heaping Tbs.)
Squash (2 heaping Tbs.)
Turnips (2 heaping Tbs.)

SALAD LIST

Tossed greens
Watercress and lettuce (romaine or Bibb or head)
Radish and watercress
Celery and cabbage
Pimiento and greens
Stuffed tomato (cottage cheese, chopped celery)
Dressing should be based on pure vegetable oil: 2 or 3 tsp. per salad,
    once daily, with seasonings to taste

DESSERT LIST

Melon, other than watermelon (¼)
Nonfat milk and diet ginger ale, half and half
Fruit cocktail, from fruit list, small portion
Whole gelatin dessert, with genuine vanilla flavor, plus small amount
    fruit from list.

At luncheon *or* dinner, one level teaspoon of butter may be used
on your vegetables. Lemon juice may be substituted for salad dressing when you wish to use two teaspoons of butter on vegetables.
Don't make this a ritual—the vegetable oils convey nutrients you
need that butter doesn't supply.

Appetite Control. Avoid soups; they tend to stimulate appetite.
Use protein tablets, available at health food stores, if appetite presses
you between meals. Choose a brand low in carbohydrate. Remember
that a little protein goes a long way in checking appetite.

Use bran tablets to keep your appetite down. Three or more 500-
milligram tablets daily have produced a sense of satiety that has
bolstered the willpower of many dieters. The number of tablets is
determined by the lessening of hunger and normalization of bowel
habits.

Reducing-diet Supplements. Eating less food means less vitamin and mineral intake, which is why supplements should be used with the reducing diet. The supplements will help to control estrogen activity and to normalize fat distribution as you lose weight. This is important for women who complain that no matter how successful they are at reducing, their dimensions shrink everywhere except where they should. Supplement the reducing diet with vitamin E, choline, inositol, and lecithin, plus vitamin B complex.

The Low-Carbohydrate Reducing Diet

I must recognize the problems of a substantial group of women who don't lose weight on the usual calorie-restricted reducing diet. These are women who have a special metabolic problem: They convert carbohydrate into fat, and they tend to store salt when they eat starches and sugars, which causes retention of fluid. The cause is the idiosyncrasy of their reaction to starches and sugars, and the remedy is to reduce the carbohydrate content of the previous reducing diet from the usual 50 percent to 25 percent, more or less (from 600 calories of carbohydrates to about 250 calories); extra protein and fat make up the difference. The diet then becomes an efficient tool for weight loss in those who have a problem with metabolizing starch and sugar and who find ordinary reducing diets ineffective.

There are several rules that must be observed if you want the regimen to be effective.

- The three meals plus three snacks aren't optional. This diet works best with frequent small meals.
- The specified frequency for the use of vegetable oil is also a must: It helps you to lose weight when you are on a low-carbohydrate diet.
- Don't try to speed up weight loss by reducing the specified

portions. You may achieve your goal at the expense of feeling tired. Stay with the recommendations for a week or two to establish your tolerance for reduced carbohydrates and then experiment with the level of starch intake to find the best compromise between feeling well and losing weight at a satisfactory pace.

- The supplements used for the preceding diet are used with this diet, too. Our goals are still control of estrogen and normalization of the distribution of the loss of body fat.

The following can be used reasonably while you are following the Low-Carbohydrate Diet:

Iodized salt
Clear broth
Unsweetened whole gelatin
Lemon
Vinegar
All spices
Sugar-free soft drinks (not cola type), but not more than 8 oz. daily
Coffee, decaffeinated

You should avoid:

Sugar-sweetened soft drinks, juices, and canned and frozen fruits that are sweetened
Vegetables packed in sugar-sweetened liquid or sauce (read labels carefully)
Foods with added corn sweetener, fructose, dextrose, glucose, honey, molasses
Cookies, cakes, crackers, pretzels, popcorn, potato and other types of chips, and other starch-sugar snack foods (eat nothing you wouldn't give to your baby or your pedigreed dog)

149

Eat a protein food—egg, meat, fish, fowl, cheese or other protein-rich dairy product—at each of the three meals and three snacks daily. Eat one egg daily, cooked as you choose. If you have a good reason for avoiding eggs, substitute two ounces of meat. Your daily intake of protein foods should be approximately ten to twelve ounces, cooked weight. Don't cheat yourself: Protein loses weight when cooked. A chop weighing five ounces raw will weigh about three ounces cooked. If you wish, substitute a quarter cup of cottage cheese for one ounce of meat; one ounce of ripened cheese for two ounces of meat.

About five teaspoons of vegetable oil daily should be used on salads. If you fall below that, take part of the oil as a supplement. This type of fat is important to the weight-loss efficiency of this type of diet. Vary your oil selections, as they differ widely in vitamin E values and content of unsaturated fats. Because of the undesirable effects of hydrogenation, I do not recommend margarine as a source of unsaturated fat. If you do use margarine, use the soft (not the stick) variety.

Two cups daily of skim milk or partially defatted buttermilk or acidophilus milk is permitted.

Eat two servings of fruit daily, chosen from the amount and types specified on the lists that follow. Canned fruits packed in syrup and frozen fruits often yield more calories from sugar than from the fruit itself.

Eat two cups of vegetables daily, chosen from those specified in the lists that follow.

You may have up to half a slice of whole-grain bread with each meal and snack. Whole-grain crackers may be substituted, weight for weight. Once daily a half slice of bread may be replaced by a half cup of beets, pumpkin, carrots, onions, peas, turnips, or winter squash. Remember, the vegetables provide fewer nutrients than the bread.

Fruit List	*Amount in One Serving*
Apple	1 small (2-in. diameter)
Applesauce	½ cup (no added sugar)
Apricots, fresh	2 medium
Apricots, dried	4 halves
Banana	½ small
Blackberries	1 cup
Blueberries	⅔ cup
Cantaloupe	¼ (6-in. diameter)
Cherries	10 large
Cranberries	1 cup
Dates	2
Figs, fresh	2 large
Figs, dried	1 small
Grapefruit	½ small
Grapefruit juice	½ cup
Grapes	12 large
Grape juice	¼ cup
Honeydew melon	⅛ medium
Mango	1 small
Nectarine	1 medium
Orange	1 small
Orange juice	½ cup
Papaya	⅓ medium
Peach	1 medium
Pear	1 small
Persimmon	½ small
Pineapple	½ cup
Pineapple juice	⅓ cup
Plums	2 medium
Prunes, dried	2 medium
Raspberries	1 cup
Rhubarb	1 cup

Strawberries	1 cup
Tangerine	1 cup
Watermelon	1 cup

Vegetable List

Asparagus	Green or wax beans
Avocado	Kale
Beet greens	Kohlrabi
Broccoli	Leeks
Brussels sprouts	Lettuce
Cabbage	Mushrooms
Celery	Mustard
Chard	Radishes
Chicory	Sauerkraut
Collards	Spinach
Cucumbers	String beans
Dandelion	Summer squash
Eggplant	Tomatoes
Endive	Tomato juice
Escarole	Turnip greens
Green pepper	Watercress

The Low-Carbohydrate Diet

BREAKFAST

Fruit or juice
1 egg
1 oz. meat or meat substitute, such as cheese or fish
½ slice whole-wheat bread with 1 tsp. soft margarine
1 cup weak tea, without sugar

MIDMORNING SNACK

1 cup skim milk, flavored, if desired, with vanilla or other sugar-
    free natural flavor
1 oz. meat or meat substitute

LUNCH

3 oz. meat (cooked weight) or meat substitute
1 serving vegetables
1 slice bread with 1 tsp. margarine
Green salad with cottonseed oil or mayonnaise (1 tsp.)
Dessert from approved selection
Weak tea or approved soft drink
NOTE: A second vegetable may be selected from the list proposed
    as bread substitutes.

MIDAFTERNOON SNACK

2 oz. meat or meat substitute
½ cup skim milk, flavored if desired
½ slice bread with small amount margarine

DINNER

3 oz. meat or substitute
Vegetable
Green salad, cottonseed oil or mayonnaise dressing
1 serving approved fruit
Approved dessert
Weak tea or other approved beverage

EVENING SNACK

½ cup skim milk, flavored if desired
1 oz. meat or meat substitute

Once you have reached your ideal weight, you leave this diet and follow the Basic Diet framework, where experience will teach you how to pattern your everyday meals to keep your weight stable.

10 | DIETARY SUPPLEMENTS

Supplements are just that. They aren't substitutes for good nutrition, but protective adjuncts to it. There is no such thing as a perfect vitamin supplement. Synthesized vitamins can lack the helpful fellow-traveling trace substances that in nature accompany the natural vitamin. Moreover, there are unknown factors in food that supplements do not contain. For this reason I caution you not to pop vitamin supplements at the expense of proper nutrition.

Supplements do provide valuable services. They cover the deficits in vitamins and minerals discarded or destroyed in food processing, offset the disadvantages of vitamins inactivated by prolonged storage or exposure to light and air, and compensate for deficits in food caused by poor soil and by fertilization aimed at quantity rather than quality. Most important to women, supplements raise your efficiency in controlling estrogen without your eating excessive amounts of food and running into a weight problem.

The Multiple Vitamin and Mineral Supplement

To assure adequate intake of the factors critical in maintaining control of estrogen activity by the liver and to make up for other nutrient deficits, you need to take a multiple vitamin and mineral supplement. A formula containing the nutrient factors in the amounts listed below would be most helpful.

MULTIPLE VITAMIN AND MINERAL SUPPLEMENT

Vitamin A: 7,500 to 10,000 units
Vitamin D: 400 units
Vitamin E: 40 units
Vitamin C: 250 mgs
B_1 (thiamine): 2 mgs
B_2 (riboflavin): 2 mgs
B_6 (pyridoxine): 3 mgs
B_{12} (cyanocobalamin): 10 mcgs
B_3 (niacinamide): 20 mgs
Pantothenic acid (d-calcium pantothenate): 15 mgs
Biotin: .3 mgs
Folic acid: 200 mcgs
Choline (bitartrate): 250 mgs
Inositol: 250 mgs
PABA (paraaminobenzoic acid): 30 mgs
Rutin (or bioflavonoids): 200 mgs
Calcium (phosphate): 250 mgs
Phosphorus (calcium phosphate): 250 mgs
Magnesium (carbonate): 200 mgs
Iron (ferrous fumarate): 15 mgs
Zinc (gluconate): 15 mgs
Copper (sulfate): 1 mg
Iodine (kelp): .15 mgs
Manganese (gluconate): 5 mgs

Chromium (chromic sulfate): 1 mg
Selenium (dioxide): .02 mgs

A dose of six tablets a day is often needed for adults and teenagers to achieve the potencies listed above. On this scale, two would be recommended for children under six, and four for children between six and twelve. Prevention is important: I would like to see nutritional protection for girls begin long before they reach puberty.

An additional supplement of vitamin E as mixed tocopherals is needed with the above formula.

The vitamin C level of the multiple formula—250 milligrams— is minimal. From 250 to 2500 milligrams daily is needed, depending on the individual. A good index of your particular vitamin C needs might be subjective criteria, such as the feeling of well-being, and objective criteria, such as your incidence of colds—their frequency, severity, and duration. Start with the amount in the multiple formula. Use a separate vitamin C supplement to raise it by 100 or 200 milligrams monthly until the optimal amount is found.

If you bruise easily adding bioflavonoids may be helpful. The quantities—in milligrams—should match those of the vitamin C supplement. There are concentrates that combine these factors.

The Vitamin B Complex Supplement

To achieve our goal of control of estrogen activity, additional supplements of vitamin B_6, inositol, and choline are needed. These are not included in sufficient potency in the multiple formula. A vitamin B complex formula should supply enough inositol to bring the intake from both supplements to at least 500 milligrams daily, the choline to 1000 milligrams, and the B_6 to 25 milligrams. Alternatively, a separate supplement of vitamin B_6 and a separate lipotropic concentrate supplying inositol, choline, and a small amount of methionine can be taken.

157

VITAMIN B COMPLEX SUPPLEMENT

Choline bitartrate	1,000 mg
Inositol (from corn)	1,000 mg
Vitamin B$_1$ (thiamine mononitrate)	5 mg
Vitamin B$_2$ (riboflavin)	5 mg
Vitamin B$_6$ (pyridoxine HCl)	5 mg
Niacinamide	50 mg
Vitamin B$_{12}$ (cobalamin conc. NF)	25 mcg
Folic acid	100 mcg
d-Biotin	30 mcg
Pantothenic acid (as calcium pantothenate)	100 mg
PABA (paraaminobenzoic acid)	30 mg

The recommendations in this book are intended for "normal" women. They are not intended for self-treatment of disease. Caution is needed because of the quirks of individual biochemistries.

- If you have cystic mastitis, uterine fibroid tumors, or endometriosis, the diet and supplements should not be used without your doctor's knowledge. This is not because there could be any adverse reactions. It simply reflects my belief that a physician who realizes the benefits of estrogen control by food will be encouraged to apply it to other women. Self-medication for any disease is unwise—you may not realize other problems are present and being neglected.
- If you're hypertensive, vitamin E must be used under medical supervision. There are a few people who suffer from hypertension whose blood pressure rises when the vitamin is first taken. They must begin with small initial doses, with the blood pressure checked regularly.
- Very high doses of vitamin C—higher than the supplementary dose suggested previously—may elevate the uric acid

level, which may mean a tendency toward gout. The effect is very rare. It may be cancelled by small amounts of folic acid, which helps to block the abnormal synthesis of uric acid.

- Allergic reactions to vitamins and minerals can occur. These are very difficult to trace as the reaction could be to the excipient used in the tablet or to a trace of a solvent used in concentrating the nutrients rather than to the vitamin itself.

APPENDIX:
FOOD ALLERGY—
THE FOOD FAMILIES

Allergy to one member of a food family indicates the strong possibility of allergy to other members of the same family. Knowing which foods are related can help you to avoid exposure to foods that may be troublemakers for you.

The foods and food families that follow are listed in two ways: In the first list individual foods are given in alphabetical order. Beside each food is a number that guides you to the family of foods in the ensuing list to which your selection belongs. In the second list food families, with all the members, are given in numerical order. The alphabetical and numerical lists will help you uncover possible allergies and also indicate safer foods. If you have absolutely no allergic reaction to a member of a food family, chances are good that you will be able to tolerate other foods in that group.

Excerpt reprinted by permission of Grosset & Dunlap from *Carlton Fredericks' New Low Blood Sugar and You,* copyright © 1969, © 1985 by Carlton Fredericks.

Food Families and Food Family Members (Alphabetical)

A

81a	abalone	68	American persimmon
80	absinthe	84	anchovy
46	acerola	84	Anchovy Family
79	acorn squash	65	angelica
1	agar	65	anise
12	agave	38	annatto
97	albacore	133	antelope
41	alfalfa	40a	apple
1	Algae	73	apple mint
63	allspice	40b	apricot
40b	almond	19	arrowroot (Maranta starch)
11	Aloe vera	16	arrowroot (Musa)
54	althaea root	19	Arrowroot Family
12	Amaryllis Family	80	artichoke flour
93	amberjack	9	Arum Family
85	American eel	11	asparagus
64	American ginseng	34	avocado

B

131	bacon	134	beef
2	baker's yeast	134	beef by-products
6	bamboo shoots	134	beef cattle
16	banana	28	beet
16	Banana Family	28	beet sugar
46	Barbados cherry	74	bell pepper
6	barley	73	bergamot
73	basil	11	Bermuda onion
112	Bass Family	23	Birch Family
53	basswood	23	birch oil
34	bay leaf	134	bison
41	bean	38	Bixa Family
129	bear	113	black bass species
66	bearberry	40c	blackberry
129	Bear Family	41	black-eyed pea
24	Beech Family	21	black pepper
24	beechnut	40c	black raspberry

Food Families and Food Family Members (Alphabetical)

B

80	black salsify	2	brewer's yeast
22	black walnut	41	broad bean
66	biueberry	36	broccoli
92	bluefish	36	Brussels sprout
92	Bluefish Family	27	buckwheat
113	bluegill	27	Buckwheat Family
80	boneset	134	buffalo
97	bonito	109	buffalofish
71	borage	6	bulgur
71	Borage Family	80	burdock root
79	Boston marrow	40d	burnet
134	Bovine Family	134	butter
40c	boysenberry	31	Buttercup Family
6	bran	79	buttercup squash
52	brandy	100	butterfish
47	Brazilian arrowroot	134	buttermilk
62	Brazil nut	22	butternut
25	breadfruit	79	butternut squash

C

36	cabbage	29	Carpetweed Family
55	cacao	1	carrageen
60	Cactus Family	65	carrot
6	cane sugar	65	Carrot Family
18	Canna Family	65	carrot syrup
79	cantaloupe	79	casaba melon
37	caper	48	cashew
37	Caper Family	48	Cashew Family
42	carambola	47	cassava
65	caraway seed	47	cassava meal
17	cardamom	34	cassia bark and buds
80	cardoon	47	castor bean
132	caribou	47	castor oil
41	carob	111	Catfish Family (freshwater)
41	carob syrup	111	catfish species
110	carp	73	catnip

36	cauliflower	6	citronella
103	caviar	45	Citrus Family
74	cayenne pepper	81c	clam
65	celeriac	73	clary
65	celery	63	clove
65	celery root	41	clover
65	celery seed and leaf	81c	cockle
80	celtuce	55	cocoa
9	ceriman	55	cocoa butter
80	chamomile	8	coconut
52	champagne	8	coconut meal
28	chard	8	coconut oil
79	chayote	79	cocozelle
134	cheese	86	cod
32	cherimoya	86	Codfish Family
40b	cherry	76	coffee
65	chervil	55	cola nut
24	chestnut	36	collards
67	chewing gum	9	colocasia arrowroot
73	chia seed	80	coltsfoot
122	chicken	36	colza shoots
41	chick-pea	71	comfrey
67	chicle	80	Composite Family
80	chicory	5	Conifer Family
74	chili pepper	65	coriander
36	Chinese cabbage	6	corn
64	Chinese ginseng	6	cornmeal
56	Chinese gooseberry	6	corn oil
14	Chinese potato	78	corn salad
79	Chinese preserving melon	6	cornstarch
7	Chinese water chestnut	6	corn sugar
24	chinquapin	6	corn syrup
11	chives	80	costmary
55	chocolate	134	cottage cheese
110	chub	54	cottonseed oil
7	chufa	41	coumarin
40a	cider	36	couve tronchuda
34	cinnamon	41	cowpea
2	citric acid	82	crab
45	citron	40a	crabapple

Food Families and Food Family Members (Alphabetical)

C

66	cranberry	79	cucumber
113	crappie	65	cumin
82	crayfish	36	curly tress
52	cream of tartar	39	currant
79	crenshaw melon	79	cushaw squash
95	croaker	86	cusk
115	Croaker Family (freshwater)	32	custard apple
95	Croaker Family (saltwater)	32	Custard-Apple Family
79	crookneck squash	4	Cycad Family
82	Crustaceans		

D

102	dab	73	dittany
80	dandelion	94	dolphin
9	dasheen	94	Dolphin Family
8	date	120	dove
8	date sugar	120	Dove Family
132	deer	52	dried "currant"
132	Deer Family	115	drum (freshwater)
40c	dewberry	95	drum (saltwater)
65	dill	119	Duck Family
56	Dillenia Family	119	duck species
65	dill seed	1	dulse

E

17	East Indian arrowroot	124	eggs, turkey
68	Ebony Family	77	elderberry
85	Eel Family	77	elderberry flowers
74	eggplant	132	elk
122	eggs, chicken	80	endive
119	eggs, duck	22	English walnut
119	eggs, goose	80	escarole
123	eggs, guinea fowl	63	eucalyptus

165

F

41	fava bean	65	Florence fennel
65	fennel	4	Florida arrowroot
41	fenugreek	102	flounder
78	fetticus	102	Flounder Family
25	fig	80	French endive
13	Fiji arrowroot	41	frijol
23	filbert	116	frog
34	filé	116	Frog Family
65	finocchio	116	frogs' legs
44	Flax Family	2	Fungi
44	flaxseed		

G

41	garbanzo	28	Goosefoot Family
27	garden sorrel	65	gotu kola
11	garlic	79	Gourd Family
134	gelatin	6	graham flour
79	gherkin	58	granadilla
5	gin	52	grape
17	ginger	52	Grape Family
17	Ginger Family	45	grapefruit
64	Ginseng Family	6	Grass Family
80	globe artichoke	61	grenadine
6	gluten flour	119	greylag goose
134	goat	74	ground-cherry
134	goat cheese	7	groundnut
134	goat ice cream	90	grouper
134	goat milk	121	Grouse Family
79	golden nugget squash	63	guava
80	goldenrod	123	guinea fowl
31	goldenseal	123	Guinea Fowl Family
41	goober	41	gum acacia
119	goose	41	gum tragacanth
39	gooseberry		

H

86	haddock	102	halibut
86	hake	131	ham

Food Families and Food Family Members (Alphabetical)

H

126	Hare Family	6	hominy grits
100	harvest fish	79	honeydew melon
100	Harvest Fish Family	77	Honeysuckle Family
23	hazelnut	25	hop
22	heartnut	73	horehound
66	Heath Family	130	horse
104	Herring Family (freshwater)	130	Horse Family
83	Herring Family (saltwater)	36	horseradish
54	hibiscus	3	horsetail
22	hickory nut	3	Horsetail Family
90	hind	79	Hubbard squash varieties
131	hog	66	huckleberry
49	Holly Family	73	hyssop

I

134	ice cream	1	Irish moss
15	Iris Family		

J

93	Jack Family	80	Jerusalem artichoke
93	jack mackerel	41	jicama
68	Japanese persimmon	5	juniper

K

68	kaki	56	kiwi berry
36	kale	36	kohlrabi
134	kefir	36	kraut
1	kelp	41	kudzu
134	kid	45	kumquat
41	kidney bean		

L

134	lactose		
134	lamb	131	lard
28	lamb's-quarters	34	Laurel Family

167

73	lavender	41	lima bean
41	lecithin	45	lime
11	leek	53	linden
41	Legume Family	53	Linden Family
45	lemon	51	litchi
73	lemon balm	82	lobster
6	lemongrass	41	locust bean
72	lemon verbena	40c	loganberry
41	lentil	40c	longberry
80	lettuce	79	loofah
41	licorice	40a	loquat
11	Lily Family	65	lovage

M

26	macadamia	6	millet
33	mace	110	Minnow Family
97	mackerel	73	Mint Family
97	Mackerel Family	6	molasses
76	Madder Family	2	mold
9	malanga	81	Mollusks
54	Mallow Family	132	moose
46	Malpighia Family	2	morel
6	malt	70	Morning Glory Family
6	maltose	25	mulberry
45	mandarin orange	25	Mulberry Family
45	mandarin tangerine	88	mullet
48	mango	88	Mullet Family
50	Maple Family	41	mung bean
50	maple sugar	45	murcot
50	maple syrup	52	muscadine
19	Maranta starch	2	mushroom
73	marjoram	108	muskellunge
98	marlin	79	muskmelon
98	Marlin Family	81c	mussel
49	maté	36	Mustard Family
74	melon pear	36	mustard greens
83	menhaden	36	mustard seed
12	mescal	134	mutton
134	milk products	63	Myrtle Family

Food Families and Food Family Members (Alphabetical)

N

43	nasturtium	96	northern scup
43	Nasturtium Family	33	nutmeg
41	navy bean	33	Nutmeg Family
40b	nectarine	2	nutritional yeast
29	New Zealand spinach		

O

6	oat	125	opossum
6	oatmeal	125	Opossum Family
87	ocean catfish	45	orange
101	ocean perch	20	Orchid Family
54	okra	73	oregano
134	oleomargarine	15	orrisroot
69	olive	42	oxalis
69	Olive Family	42	Oxalis Family
69	olive oil	81c	oyster
11	onion	80	oyster plant

P

8	palm cabbage	41	pea
8	Palm Family	40b	peach
59	papain	122	peafowl
32	papaw	41	peanut
59	papaya	41	peanut butter
59	Papaya Family	41	peanut oil
74	paprika	40a	pear
62	paradise nut	22	pecan
65	parsley	40a	pectin
65	parsnip	75	Pedalium Family
121	partridge	73	pennyroyal
58	Passionflower Family	74	pepino
58	passion fruit	74	pepper
6	patent flour	21	peppercorn
79	pattypan squash	21	Pepper Family

169

73	peppermint	61	Pomegranate Family
114	Perch Family	45	pomelo
79	Persian melon	93	pompano
122	pheasant	6	popcorn
122	Pheasant Family	35	Poppy Family
108	pickerel	35	poppy seed
120	pigeon	96	porgy
41	pigeon pea	96	Porgy Family
30	pigweed	131	pork
108	pike	131	pork gelatin
108	Pike Family	74	potato
83	pilchard	74	Potato Family
74	pimiento	82	prawn
10	pineapple	60	prickly pear
10	Pineapple Family	133	Pronghorn Family
5	pine nut	26	Protea Family
5	piñon	40b	prune
41	pinto bean	2	puffball
48	pistachio	12	pulque
102	plaice	79	pumpkin
16	plantain	113	pumpkinseed (sunfish)
40b	plum	79	pumpkin seed and meal
9	poi	40c	purple raspberry
48	poison ivy	30	purslane
48	poison oak	30	Purslane Family
48	poison sumac	16	psyllium seed
86	pollack	80	pyrethrum
61	pomegranate		

Q

122	quail	26	Queensland nut
18	Queensland arrowroot	40a	quince

R

126	rabbit	40c	raspberry
36	radish	40c	raspberry leaf
52	raisin	117	rattlesnake
11	ramp	6	raw sugar
36	rape	41	red clover

Food Families and Food Family Members (Alphabetical)

R

40c	red raspberry	80	romaine
90	red snapper	40	Rose Family
132	reindeer	101	rosefish
134	rennet	40a	rose hips
134	rennin	54	roselle
27	rhubarb	73	rosemary
6	rice	45	Rue Family
6	rice flour	121	ruffed grouse
90	rockfish	36	rutabaga
134	Rocky Mountain sheep	6	rye
104	roe		

S

80	safflower oil	80	scolymus
15	saffron	101	Scorpion Fish Family
73	sage	80	scorzonera
8	sago starch	131	scrapple
41	St.-John's-bread	86	scrod
98	sailfish	90	sea bass
105	Salmon Family	90	Sea Bass Family
105	salmon species	87	Sea Catfish Family
80	salsify	27	sea grape
80	santolina	83	sea herring
67	Sapodilla Family	95	sea trout
62	Sapucaia Family	1	seaweed
62	sapucaia nut	7	Sedge Family
83	sardine	6	semolina
11	sarsaparilla	41	senna
34	sassafras	75	sesame butter
114	sauger	75	sesame oil
131	sausage	75	sesame paste
134	sausage casing	75	sesame seed
73	savory	104	shad
39	Saxifrage Family	11	shallot
11	scallion	3	shave grass
81c	scallop	134	sheep

Food Families and Food Family Members (Alphabetical)

T

47	tapioca		41	tonka bean
9	taro		74	tree tomato
80	tarragon		6	triticale
57	tea		105	trout species
57	Tea Family		2	truffle
12	tequila		97	tuna
118	terrapin		79	turban squash
73	thyme		102	turbot
91	tilefish		124	turkey
91	Tilefish Family		124	Turkey Family
74	tobacco		17	turmeric
74	tomatillo		36	turnip
74	tomato		118	Turtle Family
86	tomcod		118	turtle species

U

36	upland cress

V

78	Valerian Family		132	venison
20	vanilla		72	Verbena Family
134	veal		41	vetch
79	vegetable spaghetti squash		40a	vinegar
79	vegetable sponge			

W

114	walleye		6	wheat
22	Walnut Family		6	wheat flour
36	watercress		6	wheat germ
79	watermelon		90	whitebait
41	wax bean		106	whitefish
95	weakfish		106	Whitefish Family
19	West Indian arrowroot		21	white pepper
128	whale		112	white perch
128	Whale Family		86	whiting

173

6	whole wheat flour	79	winter melon
6	wild rice	73	winter savory
52	wine	80	witloof chicory
40c	wineberry	76	woodruff
52	wine vinegar	80	wormwood
23	wintergreen		

Y

14	yam	114	yellow perch
14	Yam Family	49	yerba maté
14	yampi	134	yogurt
80	yarrow	40c	youngberry
9	yautia	47	yuca
112	yellow bass	11	yucca
93	yellow jack		

Z

79	zucchini

Food Families (Numerical)

PLANT

1 Algae
   agar
   carrageen (Irish Moss)
   dulse *
   kelp (seaweed)
2 Fungi
   baker's yeast ("Red Star")
   brewer's yeast (nutritional yeast)
   citric acid (*Aspergillus*)
   mold—in certain cheeses
   morel
   mushroom
   puffball
   truffle
3 Horsetail Family, Equisataceae
   shave grass * (horsetail)
4 Cycad Family, Cycadaceae
   Florida arrowroot (*Zamia*)
5 Conifer Family, Coniferae
   juniper *—used in gin
   pine nut (piñon)

* One or more plant parts (leaf, root, seed, etc.) used as a beverage.

Food Families (Numerical)

PLANT

6   Grass Family, Gramineae
     barley
       malt
       maltose
     bamboo shoots
     corn—mature
       cornmeal
       corn oil
       cornstarch
       corn sugar
       corn syrup
       hominy grits
     lemongrass
     millet
     oat
       oatmeal
     popcorn
     rice
       rice flour
     rye
     sorghum grain
       syrup
     sugarcane
       cane sugar
       molasses
       raw sugar
     sweet corn
     triticale
     wheat
       bran (semolina)
       bulgur
       flour
         gluten
         graham
         patent
       whole wheat
       wheat germ
       wild rice

7   Sedge Family, Cyperaceae
     Chinese water chestnut
     chufa (groundnut)

8   Palm Family, Palmaceae
     coconut
       coconut meal
       coconut oil
     date
       date sugar
     palm cabbage
     sago starch (*Metroxylon*)

9   Arum Family, Araceae
     ceriman (*Monstera*)
     dasheen (*Colocasia* arrowroot)
     malanga (*Xanthosoma*)
     taro (*Colocasia* arrowroot)
       poi
     yautia (*Xanthosoma*)

10   Pineapple Family, Bromeliaceae
     pineapple

11   Lily Family, Liliaceae
     Aloe vera
     asparagus
     chives
     garlic
     leek
     onion
       Bermuda
       Spanish
     ramp

175

sarsaparilla *
scallion
shallot
yucca (soap plant)
12 Amaryllis Family, Amaryl-
lidaceae
agave
    mescal
    pulque
    tequila
13 Tacca Family, Taccaceae
Fiji arrowroot (*Tacca*)
14 Yam Family, Dioscoreaceae
Chinese potato (yam)
yampi
15 Iris Family, Iridaceae
orrisroot—used in scent
saffron (*Crocus sativus*)
16 Banana Family, Musaceae
arrowroot (*Musa*)
banana
plantain
psyllium seed
17 Ginger Family, Zingiberaceae
cardamom
East Indian arrowroot
(*Curcuma*)
ginger
turmeric
18 Canna Family, Cannaceae
Queensland arrowroot
19 Arrowroot Family, Maran-
taceae
arrowroot (Maranta starch)
20 Orchid Family, Orchidaceae
vanilla

21 Pepper Family, Piperaceae
peppercorn (*Piper*)
22 Walnut Family, Juglandaceae
black walnut
butternut
English walnut
heartnut
hickory nut
pecan
23 Birch Family, Betulaceae
birch oil (wintergreen †)
filbert (hazelnut)
24 Beech Family, Fagaceae
beechnut
chestnut
chinquapin
25 Mulberry Family, Moraceae
breadfruit
fig
hop *
mulberry
26 Protea Family, Proteaceae
macadamia (Queensland
nut)
27 Buckwheat Family, Poly-
gonaceae
buckwheat
garden sorrel
rhubarb
sea grape
28 Goosefoot Family, Che-
nopodiaceae
beet
chard
lamb's-quarters

* One or more plant parts (leaf, root, seed, etc.) used as a beverage.
† Some wintergreen flavor is methyl salicylate.

Food Families (Numerical)

PLANT

spinach
sugar beet
beet sugar
tampala

29 Carpetweed Family, Aizoaceae
New Zealand spinach

30 Purslane Family, Portulacaceae
pigweed (purslane)

31 Buttercup Family, Ranunculaceae
goldenseal *

32 Custard-Apple Family, Annonaceae
cherimoya
custard apple
papaw

33 Nutmeg Family, Myristicaceae
mace
nutmeg

34 Laurel Family, Lauraceae
avocado
bay leaf
cassia bark and buds
cinnamon
sassafras *
filé—powdered leaves

35 Poppy Family, Papaveraceae
poppy seed

36 Mustard Family, Cruciferae
broccoli
Brussels sprout
cabbage
kraut
cauliflower
Chinese cabbage
collards
colza shoots
couve tronchuda
curly tress
horseradish
kale
kohlrabi
mustard greens
mustard seed
radish
rape
rutabaga (swede)
turnip
upland cress
watercress

37 Caper Family, Capparidaceae
caper

38 Bixa Family, Bixaceae
annatto—natural yellow dye

39 Saxifrage Family, Saxifragaceae
currant
gooseberry

40 Rose Family, Rosaceae
a. *pomes*
apple
cider, vinegar
pectin
crabapple
loquat
pear

* One or more plant parts (leaf, root, seed, etc.) used as a beverage.

quince
rose hips*
b. *stone fruits*
  almond
  apricot
  cherry
  peach (nectarine)
  plum (prune)
  sloe
c. *berries*
  blackberry
  boysenberry
  dewberry
  loganberry
  longberry
  raspberry*
    black
    leaf*
    purple
    red
  strawberry*
    leaf*
  wineberry
  youngberry
d. *herb*
  burnet (cucumber flavor)
41 Legume Family, Leguminosae
  alfalfa—sprouts*
  bean
    broad (vetch)
    fava
    kidney (frijol)
    lima
    mung—sprouts
    navy
    pinto
    snap
    string

wax
black-eyed pea (cowpea)
carob* (locust bean, St.-John's-bread)
  carob syrup
chick-pea (garbanzo)
fenugreek*
gum acacia
gum tragacanth
jicama
kudzu
lentil
licorice*
pea
  pigeon
  snow
peanut (goober)
  peanut butter
  peanut oil
red clover*
senna*
soybean
  lecithin
  soy flour
  soy grits
  soy milk
  soy oil
  soy sauce (tamari)
tamarind
tonka bean
  coumarin
42 Oxalis Family, Oxalidaceae
  carambola
  oxalis
43 Nasturtium Family, Tropaeolaceae
  nasturtium

*One or more plant parts (leaf, root, seed, etc.) used as a beverage.

Food Families (Numerical)

PLANT

44   Flax Family, Linaceae
      flaxseed•

45   Rue Family (Citrus Family),
      Rutaceae
      citron
      grapefruit
      kumquat
      lemon
      lime
      mandarin orange
      mandarin tangerine
      murcot
      orange
      pomelo
      tangelo
      tangerine

46   Malpighia Family, Mal-
      pighiaceae
      acerola (Barbados cherry)

47   Spurge Family, Euphor-
      biaceae
      cassava or yuca (Manihot)
       cassava meal
       castor bean
       castor oil
       tapioca (Brazilian ar-
     rowroot)

48   Cashew Family, Anacar-
      diaceae
      cashew
      mango
      pistachio
      poison ivy
      poison oak
      poison sumac

49   Holly Family, Aquifoliaceae
      maté (yerba maté)

50   Maple Family, Aceraceae
      maple sugar
      maple syrup

51   Soapberry Family, Sapin-
     daceae
      litchi

52   Grape Family, Vitaceae
      grape
       brandy
       champagne
       cream of tartar
       dried "currant"
       raisin
       wine
       wine vinegar
      muscadine

53   Linden Family, Tiliaceae
      basswood• (linden)

54   Mallow Family, Malvaceae
      althaea root•
      cottonseed oil
      hibiscus• (roselle)
      okra

55   Sterculia Family, Ster-
     culiaceae
      chocolate• (cacao)
      cocoa•
       cocoa butter
      cola nut

56   Dillenia Family, Dilleniaceae
      Chinese gooseberry (kiwi
     berry)

57   Tea Family, Theaceae
      tea•

•One or more plant parts (leaf, root, seed, etc.) used as a beverage.

58 Passionflower Family, Passifloraceae
    granadilla (passion fruit)
59 Papaya Family, Caricaceae
    papain
    papaya
60 Cactus Family, Cactaceae
    prickly pear
61 Pomegranate Family, Punicaceae
    pomegranate
    grenadine
62 Sapucaia Family, Lecythidaceae
    Brazil nut
    sapucaia nut (paradise nut)
63 Myrtle Family, Myrtaceae
    allspice (*Pimenta*)
    clove
    eucalyptus *
    guava
64 Ginseng Family, Araliaceae
    American ginseng *
    Chinese ginseng *
65 Carrot Family, Umbelliferae
    angelica
    anise
    caraway seed
    carrot
      carrot syrup
    celeriac (celery root)
    celery
      celery seed and leaf *
    chervil
    coriander
    cumin
    dill
      dill seed
    fennel *

    finocchio (Florence fennel)
    gotu kola *
    lovage *
    parsley *
    parsnip
    sweet cicely
66 Heath Family, Ericaceae
    bearberry *
    blueberry *
    cranberry
    huckleberry *
67 Sapodilla Family, Sapotaceae
    chicle (chewing gum)
68 Ebony Family, Ebonaceae
    American persimmon
    kaki (Japanese persimmon)
69 Olive Family, Oleaceae
    olive—green or ripe
    olive oil
70 Morning Glory Family, Convolvulaceae
    sweet potato
71 Borage Family, Boraginaceae (Herbs)
    borage
    comfrey—leaf and root *
72 Verbena Family, Verbenaceae
    lemon verbena *
73 Mint Family, Labiatae (Herbs)
    apple mint
    basil
    bergamot
    catnip *
    chia seed *
    clary
    dittany *
    horehound *

* One or more plant parts (leaf, root, seed, etc.) used as a beverage.

Food Families (Numerical)

PLANT

hyssop*
lavender
lemon balm*
marjoram
oregano
pennyroyal*
peppermint*
rosemary
sage
spearmint*
summer savory
thyme
winter savory

74 Potato Family, Solanaceae
eggplant
ground-cherry
pepino (melon pear)
pepper (*Capsicum*)
  bell (sweet)
  cayenne
  chili
  paprika
  pimiento
potato
tobacco
tomatillo
tomato
tree tomato

75 Pedalium Family, Pedaliaceae
sesame seed
  sesame butter
  sesame oil
  sesame paste

76 Madder Family, Rubiaceae
coffee*

woodruff

77 Honeysuckle Family, Caprifoliaceae
elderberry
  elderberry flowers*

78 Valerian Family, Valerianaceae
corn salad (fetticus)

79 Gourd Family, Cucurbitaceae
chayote
Chinese preserving melon
cucumber
  gherkin
loofah (vegetable sponge)
muskmelon
  cantaloupe
  casaba
  crenshaw
  honeydew
  Persian
  winter
pumpkin
  pumpkin seed and meal
squash
  acorn
  buttercup
  butternut
  Boston marrow
  cocozelle
  crookneck
  straightneck
  cushaw
  golden nugget
  Hubbard varieties
  pattypan

* One or more plant parts (leaf, root, seed, etc.) used as a beverage.

turban
vegetable spaghetti
zucchini
watermelon
80   Composite Family, Compositae
boneset *
burdock root *
cardoon
chamomile
chicory *
coltsfoot
costmary
dandelion
endive
escarole
globe artichoke
goldenrod *
Jerusalem artichoke
artichoke flour

lettuce
celtuce
pyrethrum
romaine
safflower oil
salsify (oyster plant)
santolina (herb)
scolymus (Spanish oyster plant)
scorzonera (black salsify)
southernwood
sunflower
sunflower seed, meal, and oil
tansy (herb)
tarragon (herb)
witloof chicory (French endive)
wormwood (absinthe)
yarrow *

ANIMAL

81   Mollusks
a. *gastropods*
abalone
snail
b. *cephalopod*
squid
c. *pelecypods*
clam
cockle
mussel
oyster
scallop
82   Crustaceans
crab
crayfish
lobster

prawn
shrimp

Saltwater Fishes

83   Herring Family
menhaden
pilchard (sardine)
sea herring
84   Anchovy Family
anchovy
85   Eel Family
American eel
86   Codfish Family
cod (scrod)
cusk

* One or more plant parts (leaf, root, seed, etc.) used as a beverage.

ANIMAL

haddock
hake
pollack
silver hake
tomcod
whiting
87 Sea Catfish Family
ocean catfish
88 Mullet Family
mullet
89 Silversides Family
silversides (whitebait)
90 Sea Bass Family
grouper
hind
red snapper
rockfish
sea bass
spotted bass
striped bass
91 Tilefish Family
tilefish
92 Bluefish Family
bluefish
93 Jack Family
amberjack
jack mackerel
pompano
yellow jack
94 Dolphin Family
dolphin
95 Croaker Family
croaker
drum
sea trout
silver perch
spot
weakfish (spotted sea trout)

96 Porgy Family
northern scup (porgy)
97 Mackerel Family
albacore
bonito
mackerel
skipjack
tuna
98 Marlin Family
marlin
sailfish
99 Swordfish Family
swordfish
100 Harvest Fish Family
butterfish
harvest fish
101 Scorpion Fish Family
rosefish (ocean perch)
102 Flounder Family
dab
flounder
halibut
plaice
sole
turbot

Freshwater Fishes

103 Sturgeon Family
sturgeon
caviar
104 Herring Family
shad
roe
105 Salmon Family
salmon species
trout species
106 Whitefish Family
whitefish

183

107 Smelt Family
 smelt
108 Pike Family
 muskellunge
 pickerel
 pike
109 Sucker Family
 buffalofish
 sucker
110 Minnow Family
 carp
 chub
111 Catfish Family
 catfish species
112 Bass Family
 white perch
 yellow bass
113 Sunfish Family
 black bass species
 bluegill
 crappie
 sunfish species
  pumpkinseed
114 Perch Family
 sauger
 walleye
 yellow perch
115 Croaker Family
 drum

Amphibians

116 Frog Family
 frog
  frogs' legs

Reptiles

117 Snake Family
 rattlesnake

118 Turtle Family
 terrapin
 turtle species

Birds

119 Duck Family
 duck species
  eggs
 goose
 greylag
  eggs
120 Dove Family
 dove
 pigeon (squab)
121 Grouse Family
 ruffed grouse (partridge)
122 Pheasant Family
 chicken
  eggs
 peafowl
 pheasant
 quail
123 Guinea Fowl Family
 guinea fowl
  eggs
124 Turkey Family
 turkey
  eggs

Mammals

125 Opossum Family
 opossum
126 Hare Family
 rabbit
127 Squirrel Family
 squirrel

ANIMAL

128   Whale Family
       whale

129   Bear Family
       bear

130   Horse Family
       horse

131   Swine Family
       hog (pork)
         bacon
         ham
         lard
         pork gelatin
         sausage
         scrapple

132   Deer Family
       caribou
       deer (venison)
       elk
       moose
       reindeer

133   Pronghorn Family
       antelope

134   Bovine Family
       beef cattle
         beef
         beef by-products
         gelatin
         margarine
         rennin (rennet)
         sausage casing
         suet
       milk products
         butter
         buttermilk
         cheese
         cottage cheese
         ice cream
         kefir
         lactose
         spray dried milk
         yogurt
       veal
     buffalo (bison)
     goat (kid)
       cheese
       ice cream
       milk
     Rocky Mountain sheep
     sheep—domestic
       lamb
       mutton

Index

187